This is the re-publication of a study originally entitled *The Deaf Child and His Family* which was a landmark in the study of early deafness. Dr Gregory's work, based on interviews with 122 mothers of deaf children under the age of six years, parallels that already done with hearing children and investigates, with the same methodology, the ways in which deaf children develop, change and are changed by their home and their wider environment. The book describes the everyday life of young deaf children and their families, looks at the deaf child's activities and daily routine, and considers the support and advice given to the parents during the child's early years. This re-publication, complete with new introduction, coincides with the publication of Dr Gregory's follow-up longitudinal study of the same cohort of families in *Deaf Young People and their Families*.

'This book gives a revealing insight into the problems of families with hearing-impaired children and is strongly to be recommended to all people involved in the education of hearing-impaired children.' 'Susan Gregory constructs a panoramic view of her subject. She displays an insight in which conciseness and compassion combine to present a balanced picture. . .' – a selection from the reviews.

Deaf Children and
Their Families

Deaf Children and
Their Families

SUSAN GREGORY

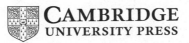

CAMBRIDGE
UNIVERSITY PRESS

Published by the Press Syndicate of the University of Cambridge
The Pitt Building, Trumpington Street, Cambridge CB2 1RP
40 West 20th Street, New York, NY 10011-4211, USA
10 Stamford Road, Oakleigh, Melbourne 3166, Australia

First published as *The Deaf Child and His Family* by George Allen & Unwin Ltd
1976
First published by Cambridge University Press 1995

Printed in Great Britain at the University Press, Cambridge

A catalogue record for this book is available from the British Library

Library of Congress cataloguing in publication data

Gregory, Susan, 1945–
[Deaf child and his family]
Deaf children and their families/Susan Gregory.
p. cm.
Originally published: The deaf child and his family. London:
Allen & Unwin, 1976. With new introd.
Includes bibliographical references and index.
ISBN 0–521–43847–0
1. Children, Deaf – Family relationships. I. Title.
HV2392.2.G74 1995
362.4′23′083 – dc20 94–45183 CIP

ISBN 0 521 43847 0 paperback

Contents

Foreword

This study of the difficulties and dilemmas encountered by a representative sample of the parents of young deaf children falls clearly within the tradition of work originating from the Child Development Research Unit at Nottingham University. It places strong emphasis on the parents' own appraisal of the task which confronts them in dealing with their own 'special' children. An insistence upon the parental perspective gives us the opportunity of understanding the development of the young deaf child in his natural setting of ordinary everyday family life, and, moreover, makes the insights of these particular parents available to others who may find themselves in a similar predicament. But these are not the only justifications for taking such a methodological approach. By using the parents of deaf children as a major resource for her investigation, Dr Gregory has drawn upon the intensive, long term, *intimate* experience of 122 mothers with 122 individual children; and this pooled experience she offers to the professional worker, whose own experience covers a variety of children but to a lesser degree of intimacy or involvement. The consequence could be a meeting-point of perspectives, so that professionals are enabled to take a new look at how they present their expertise to families, and are helped to make that expertise more relevant to their needs and hence more effective at every level. Never has this been more important that now, when there has been a deliberate shift in policy towards the progressive integration of handicapped children generally within the ordinary community. If such a policy is to be seriously and fully implemented, it follows that the family must be offered full and serious support from the moment that a diagnosis is made. It is perhaps a reflection on professional training that we sometimes assume that a problem has been tidied out of existence once it has been given a name; thus professional services on the whole tend to be better at diagnosis than at coping with the day-to-day issues which diagnosis brings into the open. Too many parents of handicapped children by the end of the first assessment find themselves suffering a double bereavement: having lost the 'normal' child they hoped for, they also lose confidence as parents because they are bereft of the information which would help them to meet the special needs of their child's handicap and thus to realise his potential.

In the case of deaf children, there is an additional reason for urgency of support. We now know that communication is gradually established between normal hearing babies and their mothers long before the child utters his first word, and that communication disorders are likely to arise whenever the pre-verbal pattern of social interaction fails to follow a normal course. The case of the deaf child can thus be viewed as an extreme instance of communication disorder in which profound and lasting damage may be done to the child's social relationships unless parents can be given skilled help at an early stage. If this analysis is correct, the work done by the peripatetic teacher with the mother of the pre-school deaf child is of enormous importance; it can in no sense be regarded as merely a holding operation until the child can be admitted to school. For the deaf child, as for the normal child, education begins in the home: he differs from the normal child in that he cannot 'pick it up naturally' from the multiplicity of learning experiences in the ordinary language-rich home, but needs special help to benefit from an often unexplained world. He cannot wait for school; and this would still be true if all the children who need it could be assured of an early place in a nursery school for the deaf.

Thus it is essential that parents should, from their very first contact with professional workers, be treated as genuine and valued partners in the therapeutic team. The implication of this is that, as professionals, we must stop hoarding our resources so defensively, and be prepared to share with parents all the information, techniques and skills which we ourselves find useful. We must stop sheltering behind jargon, and make a positive effort to make ourselves understood – and sometimes we shall no doubt find that, translated to plain English, what we had to say didn't amount to much. If we are really concerned to make parents positive forces in the remediation of their children, we shall also have to accept a shift in the professional role: we must listen to what parents have to say, make use of their special knowledge and talents, and take them into our professional confidence, so to speak, to a far greater extent than has been usual in the past.

A book like this can, we believe, give a significant impetus to the evolving of this kind of teamwork. For instance, anyone who reads between the lines of what Dr Gregory is saying will realise that there are important unresolved differences of opinion among experts as to the education of deaf children; and it is much to her credit that she has not attempted to sidestep or obscure these issues. It seems likely, however, that controversies such as these will not be resolved by more and more elaborate research on the expert level: what is really needed is a de-mystification of the professional role so that parents themselves may be allowed to contribute to a genuine collaboration. Perhaps we should ask ourselves why parental experience is the *only* kind of experience in which greater involvement is presumed to invalidate a person's opinions?

Dr Gregory begins her book by delineating the enormous communication barrier which exists between the deaf child and his mother. Everyone concerned with helping deaf children has in common the aim of breaking down this barrier. We shall succeed the better if we also acknowledge another, more subtle communication barrier – between parents and the specialists who counsel them, and who on occasion find it useful to hide behind. It should be the aim of all of us to demolish that barrier also.

John and Elizabeth Newson

Preface to the 1995 edition

This book is about young deaf children and their families. The children were all born into hearing families, the vast majority of whom knew little about deafness and had no prior experience of people who were born deaf.[1] The book looks at the young deaf children themselves and the impact of the deafness on the lives of their families. The material comes from interviews with 122 parents of deaf children in the Midlands which were carried out in the early 1970s. The book is being reissued to coincide with the publication of the follow-up study, *Deaf Young People and Their Families,* for which the same families, and the young people themselves have been interviewed.

Despite significant changes in society since the early 1970s, including developments in attitudes to deafness and the legislation that affects deaf children and adults, many of the issues and concerns of this book are as crucial now in the 1990s as they were then. The impact of the diagnosis of deafness in a child, concerns about the best way to bring up a child, and the development of language and communication are as significant now as they were a generation ago. The consequences on relationships within the family of having a deaf child, the role of the father, the effect on grandparents and relationships between siblings remain issues. Certainly, the questions asked of the parents interviewed for this book differ little from questions that might be put in the 1990s, and answers obtained then are echoed in comments made by parents of young deaf children some 20 years later.

There have, of course been changes, and the book itself could be seen as an influence in this, being the first book in this country to report research on parental, rather than professional, views of young deaf children. The book, when it was written, was one of a number of studies to give parents a voice in a way that was unusual at that time when professional accounts dominated. It was one of a series of publications arising from work carried out in the Child Development Research Unit at Nottingham University, whose Directors, John and Elizabeth Newson carried out a major study of child-rearing practices in the Midlands. More recently, the views of parents of deaf children have come increasingly to be given attention, and a number of books and articles by parents themselves have added to the discussion (see, for example, Fletcher (1987), Robinson (1987), and the accounts in Taylor and Bishop (1991), and in McCracken and Sutherland (1991)).

In this introduction, written especially for this book, I wish to look briefly at the changes within society as a whole, and at the area of deafness in particular, that impact upon the lives of deaf children and their families. I will then consider the issues in the book to examine how they are affected by this. I will also comment on the findings reported in this book in the light of current experience. My sources for this are continuing contacts with parents and their deaf children, contact with researchers in the area of deafness and recent publications on the experience of deaf children and their parents. I have also drawn on the experience of employees and of members of the National Deaf Children's Society.

However, one of the most striking things about the book to a present-day audience will not be the issues it addresses but the language it uses. In this book, deaf children are contrasted with 'normal' children throughout, with the connotations that deaf children are abnormal rather than children who are different. Deafness is described as a handicap, which would be inappropriate in present terminology. The World Health Organisation, in 1981, accepted the distinctions that had been refined by Wood, which distinguished impairment, disability and handicap. A further obvious difference is the use of sexist language throughout the book, always referring to the deaf child as 'he' unless a specific child is being discussed. This is most evidenced in the need to change the title from the original *The Deaf Child and His Family* to the less sexist *Deaf Children and Their Families*. Children from ethnic minority groups are referred to as immigrants, which was probably inaccurate then, and is inappropriate now. If the book were to be written now, the language use would be different.

The changing context

The period since the early 1970s has been one of great change in society in general, and deaf children are born into a seemingly different world.[2] The nuclear family is less robust than it was in the early 1970s, divorce is more common (rising from 5.9 per 1000 marriages in 1971 to 13.4 per 1000 marriages in 1991) and many more children grow up in families headed by a lone parent. While in 1971 less than 10% of families was headed by one parent, by the early 1991 this was 19%.

Overall, there is an impression of increasing affluence. Consumer expenditure rose in real terms by almost 70% between 1972 and 1990. Car ownership increased from just over half of all households in 1969 to two-thirds in 1991. In 1992, nearly all homes (99%) had a television, and many (72%) had a video, a rare commodity in 1971. The majority of families had washing machines (88%) and a telephone (89%). Yet, the picture is not as straightforward as this might suggest. Two reports in 1994 (Goodman and Webb, Swansea University) show the gap between the rich and the poor has increased during this period. While there has been a 50% rise in average incomes and a doubling of the income of the richest 10%, the poorest 10% are no better off than in 1967.

Employment is less stable and employment patterns are changing. Many more people are self-employed. More mothers of children under five are in full or part time work, 43% in 1991 compared with 19% in 1971. Unemployment has increased although changes in the ways of collecting information meant this is difficult to assess. In 1975 there were one million unemployed, whereas in January 1993 there were nearly three million although there have been fluctuations in the intervening period.

Major changes have been brought about by new legislation. Successive Education Acts, the National Health Service and Community Care Act and the Children Act have radically affected the provision of services with consequences for families with deaf children. Attitudes to deafness in society in general show some limited signs of change. When the parents who were interviewed for this book were interviewed some 18 years later, they were asked about this. Although most of them felt there had been some changes (65/81, 79%), only a small number (14, 17%) felt these had been major ones. For the most part, they still felt that the attitude to deafness of hearing people was one of apathy and lack of understanding. Such changes as there were, were seen to be due, in part at least, to the increasing visibility of deafness in the media, through specialist programmes and charity appeals such as Children in Need.

More specifically, within the world of deafness there have been significant and somewhat contradictory developments. The language of Deaf people, British Sign Language (BSL) has come to be recognised. In 1976, the term British Sign Language was first used for the language of signs used by deaf people. This meant that the language was no longer considered deficient, as crude mime and gesture, but as a full and proper language with all the linguistic potential of spoken languages. This legitimated its consideration as a language for families with deaf children and for education. Such recognition also contributed to the development and growth of the Deaf Community, that community of deaf people who use sign language and who see themselves as a linguistic and cultural minority group and as an active political force.

In contrast though, the development of cochlear implants has focused attention on a medical treatment for deafness. A cochlear implant is a device which stimulates the auditory nerve fibre to react to sound. It is inserted surgically, and currently is only suitable for those with little or no hearing. Although implants are only appropriate for small minority of deaf children and do not restore full hearing, the publicity that surrounds them has directed attention to the possibility of a cure of deafness, with an emphasis on normalisation and success evaluated in terms of the degree of hearing achieved.

These changes may seem to indicate that a book such as this is no longer relevant, written at a time when so many factors were different. However, it is remarkable that, despite the changes, the concerns of parents of deaf children remain essentially the same. The choices they may make may differ in detail, but the underlying issues show little variation.

Diagnosis and early support

To have a child diagnosed as deaf was, and remains a major and dramatic event in the life of most families. In the 1990s, as in the 1970s, parents talk of the difficulty of getting their suspicion taken seriously. They describe their feelings at diagnosis of shock, grief, relief, numbness and often a mixture of these. A mother writing in 1994 of the diagnosis of her then 10-year-old son, writes 'The feeling, when I was told is very difficult to put into words. It's like someone had hit me with a sledge hammer'. (Hayden, contribution to Gregory, Smith and Wells, in preparation). The impact of diagnosis should not be underestimated. In personal accounts, the time surrounding diagnosis is always described in considerable detail (see Fletcher op. cit., Robinson op. cit.). What was surprising in carrying out the interviews for the later study was that, when the

mother (or sometimes father) came to talk about the period surrounding diagnosis, they often used exactly the same words as they
had at the time of these earlier interviews. Memories of that event
had remained clear and vivid over a period of 18 or so years.

Diagnostic procedures remain similar for, despite the pressure
for early diagnosis, and the development of techniques for testing
newborn babies, these are not employed as a matter of course. The
usual practice remains to screen at 7 months, with a language
assessment in some areas at 18–21 months, and a developmental
screening at three years. As a recent report on audiological services
to children pointed out:

> As far as purely hearing services are concerned, the manner of
> delivery of services to children with hearing disorders has
> changed very little in the past 20 years apart from technical
> advances in diagnostic procedures, the sophistication of hearing
> aids and the widespread introduction of radio hearing aids.
> (Policy document of the British Association of Audiological
> Physicians, 1990)

There is an indication that, in areas where provision is good,
there may be some improvement in earlier diagnosis (Davies and
Wood, 1992) but this is not widespread, and the National Deaf
Children's Society (NDCS) still make it an issue on which they
campaign. Early diagnosis of deafness was identified by the NDCS
as one of its priorities for its golden jubilee year of 1994. They suggested certain targets.

• detecting 80% of hearing loss in both ears within the first year of
  life and 40% by the time the child is 6 months old.
• fitting hearing aids within 4 weeks of the hearing loss being confirmed.
• assessing children within four weeks of illness such as meningitis
  or difficulties at birth
• making sure that, at the age of one, all children in a district
  would have been screened to see if they are at risk of hearing
  loss.
(TALK, 1994)

Language, communication and play

A critical theme of this book is the development of language and
communication. Most parents (70%) identify it as their major con-

cern, and even more (89%) see it as the greatest problem from the child's point of view. In the 1990s, parents continue to raise this as a central issue, both in terms of how language and communication can best be developed, and their particular role and responsibility in this.

The parameters have changed somewhat, the emphasis on not using gesture has disappeared almost everywhere. In some places, advice to parents is still based on oral/aural approaches and the growth of the National Aural group (NAG) is evidence of the strength of this view. Publicity surrounding cochlear implants focuses on the use of hearing and on the development of speech although many implanted children, who previously used sign, continue to do so (Woodford, 1994). Yet the recognition of sign language, together with research showing the greater success of deaf children of deaf parents has meant that signing is now seen as a legitimate option with young deaf children and in some areas, tuition, advice and support for this is offered.

In many ways the decisions made by parents have become more complex; to sign or not to sign, to stress spoken language or sign language. The basic choices, however, remain much the same. Which approach provides the best communication with the child and the greatest potential for language development? How can good communication with all, or most, family members and friends be facilitated? Which approach will be most beneficial for the child at school and for the child's relationships in the wider hearing world?

The play of deaf children is described in some detail in this book, and it is suggested that, their activities are similar to those of hearing children, though their mother or other caregiver may intervene more. Certainly, advice to parents continues to advocate a central place for play in development with an active role for parents.

Since the publication of this book in 1976, there has been more detailed analysis of symbolic or pretend play of deaf children which suggests that, while deaf children play appropriately with pretend toys, elaborated or social symbolic play may be more difficult. It was not clear whether this was because such play required language, or could only be properly assessed through the child's comments on their own play (Gregory and Mogford, 1983).

Bringing up a deaf child

It is apparent from studies of hearing children that approaches to bringing up children have become more flexible over the past twenty or thirty years. The interviews used in this book were derived in part from those used by John and Elizabeth Newson in their studies of a cohort of children growing up in Nottingham. These interviews with parents of 1-year-old children carried out in 1958 were repeated with a new group of parents in 1986 (Newson and Lilley 1989) which gives some indication of recent changes in child-rearing practices based on parent's accounts. Overall, they indicate a more relaxed less controlling approach to children over the period. For example, in 1958 four-fifths (83%) had started toilet training by the time their children were one year old, whereas only one-fifth (21%) of the 1986 group had started toilet training by that age.

In many areas discussed in this book, including independence, meal-time behaviour and toilet training, there is little evidence of radical change apart from those consequent upon the more relaxed attitudes to child-rearing in society in general. Parents continue to encourage the developing independence of their children in a similar manner although, for both deaf and hearing children, the ability to go out of home alone has become curtailed over the past decades owing to fears of increasing traffic, but also because of the potential danger posed by other people.

Sleep and bedtime are concerns for parents in this book and continue to be issues. However, it may be that the apparent more relaxed approach to bedtimes with children as reported by Newson and Lilley (op. cit.) may remove some of the pressure from parents of deaf children feeling their children should go to bed earlier. A much smaller proportion of 1-year-old hearing babies were put to bed by 6.30 pm in the 1986 group (13%) than in the 1958 group (31%) and more than twice as many were still up after 9.30 pm (1986, 14%: 1958, 5%) This may mean that the discrepancy between deaf and hearing 4-year-old children reported in this book (p. 51) is now less significant.

Interestingly, the material on sleep patterns reported in this book was the focus of a paper published in 1978 (Tucker and McArthur, 1978). Rather than relying on the impressions given at interview by parents, their study sought to compare deaf and hearing children's sleep patterns using diary records kept over one month. The result were interesting. Deaf children seemed to need the same amount of sleep as hearing children, there was no evidence they slept less. However, they did take longer to go to sleep, almost twice as long on average. While, after 35 minutes, 90% of the hearing children were asleep, it was 55 minutes before 90% of the deaf children were asleep. The data on waking patterns was particularly revealing. There was no significant difference in the number of times of waking, or the length of time they were awake once they woke up, although averages for deaf children were higher than those for hearing children in both cases. This compares with the study in this book where it is reported that deaf children woke more often than hearing children of the same age (p. 52). It may be that, although the actual number of times is the same or similar, it seems much more because of the greater disruption caused and this accounts for the interview responses. Their paper also deals with indulgent bedtimes, but as the definition they employ is not that used in the original study, that part is ignored here.

While sleep and bedtime can be a problem for parents, it may be interesting to note that many of the parents, by the time their children were young adults, had forgotten about this. Of the 52 parents in this book reporting that their children woke in the night (p. 51), 34 were interviewed again when their sons and daughters were young adults. Of these, only 20 could recall problems with night waking.

Discipline is a major issue for parents in this book, with a focus on how to get the message across and the need for children to be well behaved. Temper tantrums, which were often seen as a response to frustration, are a particular area of concern to parents, and contemporary reports indicate that this remains so. In society in general, there has been a trend against smacking children over the past decade. However, there are indications that this has less momentum; for example, some child minders have defended their right to smack children in their care. Interestingly, the interviews with parents of one year olds indicate little change in those prepared to smack their infants in 1958 and 1986 (62% and 63%, Newson and Lilley op. cit.)

Family life

Over the past decades, fathers have been reported as taking a more active part in child care. The proportion of fathers present at the birth of their child rose dramatically from 8% to 74% between 1958 and 1986 (Newson and Lilley op. cit.) They also demonstrated that reported father participation in a number of tasks had increased over that time (bathing, taking the baby out, etc). It seems likely that this is the same with families with deaf children and certainly the professional philosophy seems to be to involve fathers more.

The consequences of having a deaf or disabled child on a marriage have been an important area of discussion, and certainly a significant number of parents in this book report it as such. While direct parallels are difficult to establish with the 1990 situation, readers may be interested to know that whether or not the marriage resulted in divorce by the time the children were grown up was not predicted by the state of the marriage as reported by the parents interviewed for this book. Those who reported that having a deaf child had driven them apart were no more likely to have separated, and those who reported that having a deaf child had made them closer were no more likely to have stayed together.

In this book, the frequency with which parents of deaf children go out and leave their child in the care of others during the day is considered, and is seen to be similar to that of parents of hearing children. The situation for parents of hearing children has changed over the past decades. In their study of 1-year-old hearing children, Newson and Lilley (op. cit.) report that parents are more likely to go out together and leave the children with babysitters or family in 1986 than in 1958. Going out together once a week increased from 22% to 30%, and more also went out sometimes, 84% compared with 60%. This trend also seems apparent in families with deaf children.

Education

A major area of change is that of education – and for a number of reasons. First, the 1981 Education Act specifies that, as far as possible, all children should be educated in local schools. This has resulted in more and more deaf children being integrated into mainstream school, and a number of schools for the deaf have closed. A direct comparison of the number in each type of school is not possible, as all the children discussed in the book had not started school at the time of the interviews. However, at the time of writing, of the five special schools available at the time of the first interviews, only two are now open and one of those is due to close. A very general comparison can be made in terms of proportion of children in each setting. At the time of the study, 76 were in school of whom 49 (64%) were in schools for the deaf or partially hearing, 19 (25%) in partially hearing units, and 8 (11%) in mainstream schools. They started school at between two and five years of age. A recent survey of the Midlands which includes the five authorities represented in the book, but others as well, gives the following figures for five year olds. Of the 256 deaf children in school, 15 (6%) were in special schools, 53 (21%) in partially hearing units and 148 (58%) in mainstream schools. The others were receiving specialist non-deaf support. (BATOD Survey, 1992, Midland Region). This is not a direct comparison, as very few deaf children in the 1990s start school before the age of five years but it does give some indication of the magnitude of the change, where previously two-thirds were in special school, and currently it is less than one in ten.

Public opinion has moved against children being sent away to boarding school at a young age – and the accounts of children being sent away at two years of age would not occur under the current system, particularly as deaf children would be less likely to attend a special school. At the time this book was originally written, one in ten attended boarding school. A survey of local boarding schools shows that there are no children under the age of six years currently boarding.

The other change is the approach to education which in the 1970s was oral, based on listening and speaking. While some children entering school in the 1990s will be offered some form of signing, the move towards integration and the impact of technology means the oral approach to education remains dominant.

Where are they now?

A major impetus for the later interviews with the families described in this book was an interest in what had happened to them, and whether things had things worked out for them. Space constraints preclude a full answer to this question, though more details are provided in the follow-up book '*Deaf Young People and Their Families*'. However, readers of this book might be interested to know the outcomes for some of the children and whether some of their fears of the parents were realised or proved to be groundless. As only a small proportion can be considered, I will only include those families who are quoted on pp. 191–193, the section in which families talk about hopes and worries for the future. Information is given wherever it is available, and if a family is omitted it is because they were not interviewed in the later study.

Isabel's parents describe their concerns about education (Girl, 3 years, severely deaf, p. 191). Isabel, in fact, attended schools for the deaf throughout her school career, going away to boarding school when she was 11 years old. This did not prevent her from later integrating into the hearing world. As an adult she worked with hearing people and had both deaf and hearing friends. In the later interview, her parents continued to express some concern about the best form of education, and queried whether they had made the right decisions. Her parents felt the education system had not demanded enough of her, and that she was understretched.

The next five parents quoted in this book express some worries about their sons and daughters, and many remained concerned, although in some instances the focus had shifted. James (Boy, 4 years, profoundly deaf, p. 192) continued to be a worry to his parents all his life. Communication within the family has always been difficult. When he grew up, his preferred communication was through sign language. The major worry within this family, however, has been his behaviour, described by one psychiatrist as hyperactive.

It was his behaviour. When he was at s.... school I just could not cope with him. He was so difficult. He would fight the others when you went out of the room. He tormented them. I took him to the psychiatrist but it was a waste of time. They couldn't talk to James. They only went on what I told them. They gave him those tablets to take to calm him down a bit. It was a complete waste of time. (Mother of James, 20 years old)

Even when he was at boarding school, his family found weekends difficult to cope with, and he was encouraged to leave home when he left school and moved into a hostel. He has had a variety of jobs in the building trade, manual labour, and has little social life. We were unable to contact him to interview him ourselves.

Samantha's mother (Girl, 4 years, profoundly deaf, p. 192) was worried about whether or not she would get married. However, as a young adult of 21 years she had a number of friends. They were mostly deaf and many were friends she made at school. She saw them mostly at weekends, and her mother felt she could be 'a bit lonely'. She had had a number of boyfriends, both deaf and hearing, but her mother commented 'They never last. She gets bored with them'. In general, she was happy with a good sense of humour. Her mother still thinks of how it might have been if she could hear 'She's so funny, if only she could hear she would have a fantastic personality'. Her mother's concerns had switched from those about getting married to what would happen if she had a baby.

I think I'd worry if Samantha had a baby. I just hope she has the money to be secure. If you have security you can cope with the rest.

Jenny's mother (Girl, 1 year, moderately deaf, p. 192) was worried that she might not get the 'natural satisfactions of life' that come from relationships. Jenny at 19 years had had many relationships, but as with Samantha they were not perceived by her mother as being stable. Her mother worried about whether in the future she would get 'a steady and stable friendship'. Jenny's preferred means of communication was Sign Supported English, the use of English plus some signs taken from British Sign Language. She had both deaf and hearing friends with whom she communicated easily. Her mother was no longer concerned about her making relationships although she was concerned that none of the friendships seemed to last. She had a hearing boyfriend while she was at school but later had a deaf boyfriend, of whom her mother disapproved although she felt it was none of her business.

She has had boyfriends. She has a boyfriend now. It wouldn't matter if the boy was deaf or hearing. She always has friends but they are always changing. There is no stability there.

However, in common with a number of the young people, Jenny's description of the situation was different. She felt she had a good social life with lots of friends and described meeting them most evenings as she hated to be on her own. Her current partnership was a serious relationship and she explained that her current boyfriend wanted to marry her in three months but that she wanted to wait for a year. This discrepancy between parents and young people was not unusual and we suggest in *Deaf Young People and Their Families* that it could arise from different perceptions of the situation.

The mothers of both Ann (Girl, 4 years, profoundly deaf, p. 192) and Jean (Girl, 3 years, profoundly deaf, p. 193) were worried about their daughters' communication and the consequences for relationships, and for both of them the worries persisted. Both the young people were interviewed for the later research but were among those whose responses could not be used in the quantitative analysis because of difficulties in communication. (This is discussed in more detail in *Deaf Young People and Their Families*). However, for both of them, restricted opportunities to communicate seemed to contribute to their communication problems. Ann, as she grew up, was excluded from many family events, she cooked for herself and ate in her own room, she only knew of her mother's remarriage, when her stepfather moved in. She seemed to have little opportunities for any social life, although she had a boyfriend she had met at school. He lived some considerable distance away but visited regularly and she planned to go and live with him in the future. Jean's mother continued to feel sorry for Jean and to worry about her. She was disappointed in the lack of achievement but there seemed to be few opportunities for Jean to achieve. When interviewing Jean the interviewer commented 'Her comprehension of question was poor, but I felt this was partly due to the lack of real communication at home and not having positive experience in relation to her own peer group'. Her mother's worries at the later interview were reflected in her comment then:

> *Being left on her own. We have made provision if anything happened to us. . . She is going to be devastated. It's the fact of having to leave her one day without knowing she's properly adjusted to cope. Mothers always worry about their children whether they are deaf or not.*

In these instances, it is difficult to know whether the later lack of linguistic competence was due to problems with communication to which the mothers were sensitive, and which was implicit in their descriptions, or whether the low expectations of the family early on had consequences for their daughters development.

The parents of both Paula (Girl, 6 years, profoundly deaf, p. 193) and Jean (Girl, 6 years, moderately deaf, p. 193) describe their hopes for the future. Paula was 24 at the time of the second interviews and used BSL to communicate. She had a job, and an active social life with both deaf and hearing friends. When her mother was asked in the later interview about her hopes for the future, she implied it was already happening.

> *Oh, for her to have a happy life, full employment, to be fulfilled and just enjoy herself. What is actually going on. No different actually, no different at all.*

Carol's life had not been without problems as she grew up, and in particular her education has been interrupted. At the time of the second interviews she was 23 years old, and used speech to communicate, although many of her friends were deaf and she was going to classes to learn BSL. She had left school with 4 GSCEs although was probably potentially capable of a lot more. At the time of the interviews she seemed more settled. Her mother said:

> *You need to be very guarded about expecting your child to achieve what all children achieve. I think this is the mistake we made. And we were misled to some extent by some of the specialists that we saw in thinking that Carol was super-intelligent. We were given this impression several times, weren't we? We were led to believe she had got a high IQ, was going to be a super-achiever, which was wrong. . . I think we pushed her more than we should have done. I think she is very intelligent in some ways, but not in an academic way, definitely not.*

At the end of this interview the parents reflected on the interview itself.

> *Mother: It is upsetting going through it all again. . . It is a bit shattering. There are times when you talk to people like you, when you realise just what you have achieved, in spite of all the things that are still wrong and that you are still not happy about. We have achieved a lot.*
> *Father: Yes, and what **Carol** has achieved. It is so easy to criticise and compare and think what might be better and overlook what she has gone through, what she has achieved in spite of it all.*

NOTES

1. Although all the families in this study were hearing parents of deaf children, a parallel study using the same interview schedule has been carried out with deaf parents and their deaf children (Hartley, 1988).
2. Except where indicated otherwise, the data reported is from the Central Statistical Office (*Social Trends*, Vol. 24, HMSO 1994).

REFERENCES

BATOD (1992), 'BATOD Survey 1992 Midland Region,' *Association magazine, British Association of Teachers of the Deaf,* January 1993
British Association of Audiological Physicians (1990), *Paediatric Audiological Medicine* (British Association of Audiological Physicians, Cardiff)
Davis A.C. and Wood, S. (1992), 'The epidemiology of childhood learning impairments: factors relevant to planning of services', *British Journal of Audiology*, Vol. 26, pp. 77–91
Fletcher, L. (1987), *A Language for Ben* (Souvenir Press, London)

Goodman, A. and Webb, S. (1994), *For Richer, for Poorer* (Institute of Fiscal Studies, London)

Gregory, S. and Mogford G. (1983), 'The development of symbolic skills in young deaf children' in Rogers, D.R. and Slobada, J.A. (ed.) *The Acquisition of Symbolic Skills* (Plenum Press, London)

Hartley, G. (1988), 'Aspects of the homecare of deaf children', unpublished PhD thesis (University of Nottingham).

Hayden, A. (in preparation) 'Scott', in S. Gregory, S. Smith and A. Wells, (eds) *Bilingual Education and Deaf Children*, to be published by Multilingual Matters, Clevedon.

McCracken, W. and Sutherland, H. (1991), *Deaf Ability not Disability* (Wayside Books, Clevedon)

Newson, J. and Lilley, J. (1989), 'Continuity and change in patterns of infant care during the first year', paper presented to the La Leche League National Conference, Oxford, September 1989

Robinson, K. (1987), *Children of Silence* (Gollancz Press, London) (reissued, with a new foreword, 1991, Penguin Books, Harmondsworth)

Swansea University (1994), *Winners and Losers* (Department of Economics, Swansea University)

Talk (1994), 'Quality standards in paediatric audiology', *Talk, 152.*

Taylor, G. and Bishop, J. (eds) (1991) *Being Deaf* (Pinter Publishers, London)

Tucker, I. and McArthur (1978), 'The sleep patterns of pre-school hearing impaired children', *Journal of The British Association of Teachers of the Deaf*, Vol. 2, No. 1

Wood, P. (1981), *International Classification of Impairments, Disabilities and Handicaps* (World Health Organisation, Geneva)

Woodford, D. (1994), 'An investigation into children with cochlear implants', carried out on behalf of the British Deaf Association (The British Deaf Association, Carlisle)

Acknowledgements

This study would not have been possible without the financial support of the National Deaf Children's Society. The Society exists to promote the welfare of all deaf children. To quote from their policy statement:

> The National Deaf Children's Society which welcomes as members Parents, Teachers of the Deaf, Otologists, Missioners and ALL actively concerned with the welfare of deaf children, exists to promote and ensure for the children the maximum benefits and happiness from:
> (a) Their home environment
> (b) Educational facilities
> (c) The cooperation of the general public.

The society provides an advisory service to parents, and circulates a quarterly magazine, *Talk*, as well as other free literature.

It must be made clear at the outset that all the views expressed in this book are those of the author, and do not necessarily reflect the policy of the National Deaf Children's Society.

The studies by John and Elizabeth Newson, of normal children growing up in Nottingham, form an essential background to this book. Their experience and interest was of immense value to me in carrying out this research, and I should like to express my personal gratitude to them for their guidance and support.

The idea for a study of deaf children to parallel the work with normal children was proposed by the late Professor M. M. Lewis, and I am grateful to him for his help and encouragement in the initial stages of the research. Mr Michael Reed advised me on various aspects of deafness in the final stages of the project, and I am particularly grateful to him for reading through my manuscript, and for his useful criticisms and comments.

I should also like to thank the East Midlands Regional Association of the National Deaf Children's Society, and in particular their Chairman, Mr P. Knighton, and their Welfare Secretary,

ACKNOWLEDGEMENTS   xxix

Mrs B. Howard, for their support and continuing interest in this study.

I am also indebted to those schools who welcomed me in the early stages of the research and gave me first-hand experience with deaf children. In particular I should like to thank Mr J. R. W. French and the staff and pupils of the Ewing School for the Deaf, Nottingham, and Mr J. M. Ashton and Mrs J. L. Colledge and the pupils of the Aldecar C.I. School Partially Hearing Unit. I should also like to thank Mr D. Grossman, Senior Peripatetic Teacher, Herts, for his help in arranging the pilot study.

My thanks also go to Miss M. Plackett of the Library of the Royal National Insitute for the Deaf for her assistance, and to Miss E. M. Stewart for her secretarial services.

Finally, my sincere gratitude goes to the 122 mothers who described so vividly their experiences with their own deaf children, and those words form a vital part of this report. It is to them that this book is dedicated.

Chapter 1

The Handicap of Deafness

Without knowing a deaf child it is very difficult to comprehend what it is like to have one in the family. The deaf child looks normal, and yet his handicap is very real. For those people who have never encountered a young deaf child it is hard to understand how much difference it can make. One might think of what a person misses who cannot hear music, or church bells, or the birds sing. One might think of some of the practical problems of having a small deaf child, that he does not hear cars coming, a horn hooting; that one cannot call out to warn of danger and so one has to keep him close. But it is not these things that constitute the real problem. Life is impoverished without the joy that various sounds can bring, and there are situations which can be dangerous for someone who cannot hear; but there are greater problems than these. It is learning to understand other people, and to talk to them, that is the real area of difficulty.

A normal hearing child learns to talk because he is constantly being talked to. He comes to realise that the sounds made by the human voice are of special significance. How difficult it is, though, for the child who cannot hear the human voice, or who can only hear one or two sounds. Without special teaching he will not learn to understand other people, or to talk himself. Even with special teaching, one can never provide the vast experience the hearing child has of spoken communication. The deaf child with limited, or even no understanding of what is said to him and not being able to talk himself can be cut off in many ways from what goes on around him. In essence then, this is the problem: communication.

Helen Keller, probably the most famous deaf-blind person of our age, said of the handicap of deafness:

The problems of deafness are deeper and more complex, if not more important than those of blindness. Deafness is a much worse misfortune. For it means the loss of the most vital stimulus – the sound of the voice that brings language, sets thoughts astir, and keeps us in the intellectual company of man.[1]

More recently, during a television programme[2] a man deaf from birth said:

Blindness cuts people off from things, deafness cuts people off from other people.

When the mothers were interviewed for this research, they were asked what they felt their greatest problem was in coping with their own deaf child. Seventy-six per cent of them gave answers indicating problems that arose from difficulties in communicating. When asked what they felt was the greatest problem from the child's point of view, 89 per cent replied that it was communication. Most of the remaining answers were problems specific to a particular child, and no one other problem was mentioned more than three times. Communication with, and for, the deaf child is by far and away the greatest problem.[3]

What does this mean in real terms? What do mothers need to be able to communicate to their children under six? Not being able to explain things can make it very difficult to get across to the child what he is, and what he is not, permitted to do.

Boy, 5 years
I think trying to tell him what is right and what he should do and what he shouldn't do – it's very difficult. He can't understand why it's wrong – you see. Like he'll see a lady in the garden, and he'll see that lady pick some flowers and of course he thinks he can do the same. It's her garden, you know, and this is our garden, you can't tell him right from wrong at the moment. The thing is getting through to him. It's very frustrating for yourself you know. To me it wears me out sometimes, it really wears me out trying to get through to him at times, it really does.

Even when it is possible to get the message across, it often has to be just a 'No' with no possibility of explaining to the child why. This makes some mothers feel they are somehow cheating their children.

Boy, 4 years
I mean you can't say, like when Janet (his sister) gets older, we'll say 'Now you won't touch the fire because it will burn.

Nasty. Hurts.' But all you say to Stephen is say 'No' and that's it. You just can't explain why. It's horrible.

Girl, 2 years
You can't temper it. It's either a definite yes or a definite no, which I find very difficult. That is about the most difficult thing for me.

Without any explanation, life may seem to be one arbitrary rule after another. One very common way of getting across to a child that what he is doing is wrong is the formula 'If you do that again I'll . . .' The child knows what he is doing is wrong and knows what the consequences will be if he does it again. For many parents it seems totally unfair to punish a child for something he does not know is wrong, and yet it may be impossible to warn a deaf child in this way.

Girl, 3 years
I think that, because she can't hear you can't tell her the first time. Like with a normal child you can say 'You do this again and I'll smack you next time you do it', but with Wendy, you've either got to let her get away with it, else turn away. She didn't use to look at me so I couldn't tell by expression on my face so it had to be a tap.

Another important area is persuading the child to wait for something. A busy mother is not always able to stop what she is doing to mend a broken car, or find a missing piece of a puzzle. Small children are impatient at the best of times, if 'Wait a minute' seems like 'No' to them, it may be just too much.

Girl, 4 years
The hardest thing to teach her is when she's got to wait a minute – to wait. She's got to rush here, and rush there. She can't understand 'In a minute'. If she wants something, she wants it there and then, not two or three minutes later.

For the next little boy, his desperation was because if his mother did not stop immediately he did not feel he was understood.

Boy, 4 years
Well I have to stop, because he gets terribly agitated, and he feels that I can't hear him, I think. I'll say 'In a minute, Peter, in a minute', or something like that and he'll fall on the floor because he seems to think he hasn't got across to me I think. He gets terribly upset so I have to stop.

The boot may be on the other foot, it may be that a mother needs to get a child to hurry. This is difficult with many normal children, but may be exacerbated if reasons cannot be given.

Boy, 4 years
He tends to get involved, and then the problem is communicating to him the urgency of the matter in hand – we may have arranged to go shopping on a Saturday morning. He'll accept it, but it's difficult. Having explained it to him and made sure he's understood, because if you whip him away and he hasn't understood you've still got a battle to fight. You have to make your peace there and then.

While many mothers of deaf children can explain to hurry, or to wait just a minute in the immediate situation, when the waiting extends farther into the future, it may be more difficult. One important thing that mothers need to get across is 'soon' or 'later', the idea that something will not happen now, but will in the future. To explain to a child that he cannot go out now but will be able to after dinner is another example.

Boy, nearly 3 years
It's things in the future that are difficult to get through to him, like 'After dinner we'll go out' sort of thing, he only understands things that we're doing at the moment, and as I say you can't promise him anything.

Once out playing, or at a friend's house, a small child often does not want to come home, and often it is the reassurance that he can go back another time which induces him to come away. But it may not be possible to get this across to the deaf child.

Boy, 4 years
When we're going somewhere, and he's really enjoying himself, and say we've got to go and it's late and the baby needs to be fed. Then you can't say to him 'Come on Stephen, we've got to go home now. We can come back tomorrow.' You've just got to say 'Come on Stephen, going now.' And he doesn't want to go. It's because you can't say why he can't do things and why he has to do things that really hurts me. You can't say, like when we go to Robert's to play, 'We're going now, we'll come back tomorrow. Just one more day and we'll come back', or when we take him to the park 'We'll come another day.' To him we're going and we're never going there again as far as he's concerned. You know, you can't explain that you will go back again.

Looking forward to Christmas, birthdays, holidays is an exciting part of a young child's life, but to explain to a deaf child that something exciting is going to happen can be difficult.

Girl, 5 years
If it's sort of a Santa Claus is coming thing it's ever such a job. See we've had some Christmas cards come to send off and she thinks it's a birthday, you know. Anything in the distance is difficult.

Even when a mother can get across that something will happen in the future, trying to recall the past can be difficult.

Girl, 4 years
You can say something will happen in the future, but you can't say 'Do you remember what happened the other day?' – she can't think backwards. It leads to confusion. The other day my mother was here, and last summer she took them to the seaside with a friend of hers who also took two grandchildren. One of these children was called Joan, and my mother came to lunch and we were eating and Brenda wouldn't eat her dinner and Mum said 'Try to say to her – do you remember at Skegness we used to have a race and Brenda and Joan would race to finish.' We tried to get this over to Brenda but Brenda thought we meant we were going to Skegness again, and after lunch we found she'd got her suitcase packed and her dolls all ready to go – which was awful. Very upset, and I had to raid my Christmas presents and so on. She can't . . . I've never managed to get over to her 'do you remember . . .' even yesterday. She thinks whatever happened that you're saying you're going to do it now.

Telling Daddy about the day, when he comes in from work, is a way of including Daddy in the day's events, for many hearing children.

Girl 4 years
She's just beginning to understand that we're going to do things tomorrow. But we can't talk about things she has done. I often try to say to her, 'Remember to tell Daddy', with things we've done. When Daddy comes I say 'What do you remember'? She doesn't know – I think she knows I mean she should talk about it, I don't think she can – she does remember the things but she doesn't understand you want her to tell someone what she did. You can't really talk a lot about things she did because she thinks that you're saying that she's going to do them again.

At first sight, not being able to talk about the past and the future may not seem an overwhelming problem, but it is these sort of conversations that enable a child to see life as continuous and structured. Christmas Day, instead of being a climax of wrapping presents and putting up decorations, can seem an isolated day. More important, if the deaf child is out playing, or at school, and cannot tell his mother about what he has been doing, his day, for him, may become divided into isolated segments. Communication is not just the imparting of information but has a wider significance in that it is a way of maintaining contact and continuity.

Of course, not all the problems mentioned above apply to all young deaf children. Many deaf children do learn to talk, but it can be a very slow process. In the 122 deaf children in this sample only a quarter could put two or more words together to make a simple sentence. A further quarter, while not putting words together at all, had a vocabulary of more than five words. This means that half the group had a vocabulary of five words or less, and half of these, a quarter of the total group, could not use the spoken language at all to communicate. Of course, the older the child the more likely he was to be able to use the spoken language. (See Table 1.1.)

Age	Language Used			
	sentences	over six words (not sentences)	five or less words	none
2·0–3·5 years	11% (3)	19% (5)	33% (9)	37% (10)
3·6–4·11 years	21% (9)	38% (16)	21% (9)	19% (8)
5·0+ years	56% (19)	29% (10)	12% (4)	3% (1)
Total sample	25% (31)	25% (31)	25% (31)	24% (29)

Table 1.1   Language used by the deaf child, by age
(this excludes children under 2 years and immigrant children)

When we come to consider how much of the spoken language a child can understand we face a problem. It is very difficult to determine how much a child can understand because when one speaks to a child the spoken word is not the only clue as to what is going on. Facial expression, gesture, and of course the situation itself all give clues as to the meaning of what is being said. Instead, then, of asking what the child could understand, we asked *who* the child could understand. A deaf child who can understand almost anyone who talks to him, providing, of course, they make sure that they are in a good light, and are speaking clearly, and the child is attending to them, has some grasp of the spoken language. Only 30 per cent (36) of the children could understand anyone who spoke to them. A further 27 per cent (33) could understand people they knew. But 19 per cent (23) could not understand anyone at all, and 25 per cent (30) could only understand their mothers. This means that 44 per cent of the children were cut off from conversation with the people they came into daily contact with (excluding their mothers). (See Table 1.2 for a breakdown of these figures by age.)

Age	People Understood			
	almost anyone	relations and friends	mother only	no one
2·0–3·5 years	22% (6)	15% (4)	37% (10)	26% (7)
3·6–4·11 years	29% (12)	38% (16)	19% (8)	14% (6)
5·0 years	50% (17)	32% (11)	17% (6)	0 (0)
Total sample	30% (36)	27% (33)	25% (30)	19% (23)

Table 1.2 People whose language is understood by the deaf child, by age
(this excludes children under 2 years and immigrant children)

The general reader might well be asking why there is all this emphasis on spoken language – surely the deaf communicate by signs. The usual image of a deaf person is someone who gesticulates, who speaks with his hands. But current educational practice with very young deaf children discourages the use of any form of sign language.[4] The ultimate aim is to get children integrated into normal society, to be able to communicate with hearing people. It is felt by many that this is best achieved by the intensive use of language. Certainly there had been no attempt with any of the children under consideration here to teach signs. Of course there was a great deal of communication using gesture, but this mostly took the form of an exaggerated version of the normal gesture of communication and could only be used to get across simple ideas. It consisted mainly of pointing and miming, and had nothing like the range of possibilities for communication that the formal sign language used by many deaf adults has.

The mothers were asked how they usually communicated with

their deaf children. Some mothers relied almost exclusively on
gesture.

Girl, nearly 2 years
If she's not looking at me I touch her face and then point at what
I want, and get through to her that way.

Others combined gesture and speech in various ways.

Boy, 4 years
Well we find that we've got hand gestures and signals and speech.
We use the speech as well but we use the hand signals to get it
over to him.

Girl, 2 years
I talk to her, and then if she doesn't understand I put in a few
signs. But quite obviously any young child uses a lot of signs
at this age, as well as talking, and so I haven't stopped her. I
think it's all right for her to – and speech will come.

Boy, 4 years
We always try and get him facing us. We try and tell him without
the actions if we can.

Other mothers were able to rely almost totally on speech.

Boy, 3 years
We just talk to him normally. It just comes natural. We always
just touch him and then talk to him.

Overall, when the mothers were asked how they usually communicated with their deaf child, 28 per cent (34) said they
usually communicated by talking to him, albeit more slowly and
clearly than to a hearing child. On the other hand 30 per cent (36)
of the mothers did not use speech but normally used gestures and
pointing. The remainder used a combination of gesture and speech.
As one might expect, the older the child, the more likely the mother
was to use speech as the medium for communication.

The mothers were also asked how their deaf child communicated
with them. Just over half the children, 57 per cent (68), relied
exclusively on gesture, showing or pointing.

Boy, 4 years
He uses his hands. He does a lot of miming. He doesn't seem to
bother with speaking now. He sort of mimes it to you.

Boy, 4 years
Mostly by showing me. He'll come and show me, then do a few
of his signals.

Girl, nearly 2 years
She brrs to get attention, and then she points. If she wants me to look she'll point to her hand and then point to something, so I've got to look.

Boy, 3 years
He just takes me by the hands and leads me to wherever it is he wants to go, and then points. That's his only way.

Some children had very ingenious ways of communicating without using speech.

Boy, 5 years
He usually explains with his hands, and tries to say the word of what it is. If it's something in particular he's looking for, if he remembers that it's in a book he'll fetch the book and he'll show me what he's looking for, and then I usually know straight away. For anything he eats he'll go (points to mouth) like that, and if he wants to go to the toilet he holds himself. If he wants to go to bed he does this (points upstairs).

Girl, 4 years
Well, if she wants a drink she usually goes like that, or points if she wants a biscuit, if she wants anything in a cupboard she usually points. If she wants to go to the toilet she points to herself or holds herself, but she gets through all right.

Twenty-four of the children used speech and gesture, mainly resorting to gesture when they could not get the message across by speaking.

Boy, 3 years
If he can't make me understand by saying, he will then show me what he wants. In fact if I can't understand him I will say 'Well you show Mummy.'

Girl, 3 years
Mainly language – the odd thing she'll try and tell you first, and if I just can't understand she'll show me. When she's showing you, you know what it is. There's no problem in communicating.

Boy, 3 years
Yes it's one of those things. We can understand what he's on about but you wouldn't understand him but we can. Sometimes he might show you, other times he'll try to tell you with actions.

Girl, 4 years
She tries to say the words she knows but she also mimes. She's

taught a lot of mime and gesture at school and she uses these and school never tells us what they mean so Nicky teaches us. She's quite good – she tells us what she means.

Only 24 per cent (28) of the whole group normally communicated by speech. For those children who did use speech as a means of communication, it was felt by many of them to be a very real achievement if they did manage to make themselves understood.

Boy, 3 years
(Q136: Is he pleased when you understand, or does he take it for granted?)
Yes. Well if it's something new he's saying he seems to know it's new and gets ever so excited.
(Q: He doesn't take it for granted you'll understand?)
If it's things he's said over and over again – yes, but if it's new – no.

Boy, 4 years
(Q136: Is he pleased when you understand, or does he take it for granted?)
He does show pleasure, because we obviously reiterate what he's said for him to say yes to – so he knows that we've understood and this sort of thing. He will say 'Oh – that's right.' He'll be quite open and quite joyful about it – it may take three or four tellings.

For the majority of children, trying to communicate was at times frustrating. Such gesture as they used was inadequate for communicating more than very simple ideas. These children wanted to talk but often they could not. For many of them their attempts to speak just did not work.

Girl, 5 years
She tends to move her mouth and there's no voice coming out and yet she thinks she's talking.

Girl, 2 years
She wants to talk to you, you can see she does, but she just doesn't know how.

Girl, 4 years
She wants to use the word, but it can't come.

Girl, 3 years
I think, if only she could talk. She gets very excited and she can't tell you. She can't tell you that she's pleased with it. She

shouts and she screams. When I say she screams it's not temper. It's because she's overjoyed with something, but she can't explain herself.

And for some, their attempts to speak actually inhibited communication.

Boy, 3 years
When he's speaking to me, and I say 'What's that you say baby?' he'll pull his mouth wide open, you know, and his eyes will go and it's worse then, you know. He can't say anything at all. He'll just take my hand and show me what he wants. He tries that hard to make himself understood, the words come out worse.

If we look at the mode of communication by age (Table 1.3) it seems apparent that there is a shift to communication by the spoken word between the 3·6–4·11-year-old group and the children over 5 years.

It thus seems that the transition to communication by the spoken word only gathers impetus after the age of 3½ for the young deaf child, whereas hearing children increasingly use the spoken word from the age of 2 years. Although the proportion of children using the spoken word doubles between the 3½–5 age group and the over-5s, still at 5 years less than half the deaf children are using the spoken word as their mode of communication. Even at 5 years, a third of the group are still relying totally on gesture to communicate.

Age		Mode of Communication		
		spoken word	gesture	both
2·0–3·5	years	11% (3)	67% (18)	22% (6)
3·6–4·11	years	21% (9)	62% (26)	17% (7)
5+	years	44% (15)	32% (11)	23% (8)

Table 1.3 Mode of communication of young deaf children broken down by age (excludes children under 2 years and immigrant children)

Hence it is clear that the problem of communication is a very real one. The children who were communicating by signs and those communicating by gesturing were incapable of getting across anything like the range of a normal child. Clearly they have the feelings, preferences of a normal child, but communication by gesture tends to be 'black and white' – lacking subtlety and qualification and being blunt and to the point. This issue will be seen to lie at the root of most of the other problems that are described and discussed in later chapters.

Until now, in this book, deafness has been discussed as if it was a simple handicap – simple in the sense that a deaf child is just a child who cannot hear. Of course this is not the case. There are various degrees of hearing ranging from normal hearing (normal for humans) to total deafness, though in fact total deafness is very rare. In the majority of cases described in this book, the child has some hearing, although it might only be a small amount.

Some attempt was made at the interview to derive an assessment of the child's functional hearing, i.e. the range of sounds he would respond to in his day-to-day life. It must be made clear that this is not purely a description of the child's hearing loss but will depend on other things as well: his level of intelligence, his past experience of sounds, the use to which he puts his hearing aid if he has one. While not being an assessment of hearing loss *per se*, it seems the most realistic approach to take with young chilen. With older children and adults it is usually possible to obtain an audiogram of response to pure tones in a clinic setting, which comes close to providing an indication of the true degree of hearing loss, but this is often not possible with small children. At this age, and particularly with children under 3 years, it is very difficult to get an accurate assessment of how much the child can hear. The assessments given here then, while basically reflecting a child's hearing loss, must not be taken to be an absolute measure.

In assessing the hearing loss of a child, all relevant answers were used, although special attention was paid to the following questions.

6 [5] I wonder if we can get an idea of how deaf N is. Can he hear anything at all?

7   Can he hear if you shout (or talk normally) close to him when he's not wearing his hearing aid?
... and with his aid?

8   Does he take much notice of sounds? (Note any in particular)

17   Have you been told how deaf he is? If yes: Do you know the results of his last hearing test?

19   Do you know if his hearing has got better or worse?

104   If you needed to stop him doing something,
       is there any way you can get his attention
       without actually going over to him?
       If yes: How?

After the interview, the interviewer noted down all incidents of communication between the child and anyone else during the interview.

On the basis of all the various evidence, a description was then written of the child's hearing. For the purposes of scoring, the hearing was classified into the categories shown in Table 1.4.

Category	%
0 No response to sound with or without aid	5
For children with aids	
1 Response to few loud noises only	14
2 Limited response to voice when attending	30
3 Response to voice even when not attending	30
4 Near to normal responses	9
For children without aids	
5 Responses to loud noises only	0
6 Response to voice when attending	2
7 Response to voice even when not attending	2
8 Near to normal responses	2
9 Not known[a]	7

Table 1.4 Incidence of different degrees of deafness in this sample

[a] See the end of the guided interview schedule, Appendix I, for the hearing assessment key.

It is not necessarily true that this distribution is typical of the deaf population in general, or even the population of young deaf children. In order for a child to be included in this sample, deafness had to be diagnosed, and many cases of deafness are not picked up until the child reaches school-age. For this reason one would expect this sample to be weighted in favour of the more severely deaf, for these are the ones most likely to be diagnosed at this early age.

Throughout the book quotes taken from the tapes of the interviews are given to provide illustrations.[6] In order to provide a context for each quote it is labelled with a description of the child to whom it applies in terms of age, sex and hearing loss. The hearing loss is described by the following terms.

profoundly deaf: little or no response to sound, no response to the human voice
(Categories 0, 1, 5 — 19% of sample)

severely deaf: response to human voice but limited to situations when the child is attending
(Categories 2, 6 – 32% of sample)

moderately deaf: response to voice in favourable situations
(Categories 3, 7 – 32% of sample)

partially hearing: near to normal responses, though hearing loss constitutes a handicap
(Categories 4, 8 – 11% of sample)

not known: hearing loss not possible to assess, either because the child is very young or presents particular problems
(Category 9 – 7% of sample)

The following examples may make these categories clearer.

Collette is $4\frac{1}{2}$ years old and profoundly deaf. Occasionally she seems to hear very loud noises, but not consistently, and she never responds to the human voice. She was a premature baby, only weighing just over 3lb at birth and her deafness is attributed to this. She was kept under observation for her first year although deafness was not confirmed until she was 2 years old, as originally her slowness in speech and lack of response was thought to be due to mental retardation. She is now thought to be of average intelligence.

She does not say any words or understand anything that is said to her, although she is now beginning to look at people's lips when they speak. She communicates by gestures alone, and her mother finds not being able to explain things to Collette the biggest problem. To get Collette's attention her mother stamps on the floor and sometimes Collette will respond to the vibrations, but it is impossible to rely on this.

She has a hearing aid which she was reluctant to wear at first but now wears all the time. There is no peripatetic service[7] in her area and since the age of 3 she has been a weekly boarder at a school for the deaf.

Emily is 2 years old and severely deaf. She seems to hear one or two loud noises: a cuckoo clock, aeroplanes, the door bell and a whistle. She occasionally responds to a person shouting to her, but not consistently.

The cause of her deafness is unknown. She passed a routine hearing assessment test at 8 months, but at 12 months her mother was worried as she showed no signs of starting to talk. Further examination showed Emily to be severely deaf and this diagnosis was confirmed at 15 months.

She has a hearing aid which does not seem to help her much, and which she is reluctant to wear although she generally wears it for some time each day. She communicates by gestures but is beginning to watch people's lips when they speak to her. Not being able to get her attention by calling her, but having to go over to her every time she is wanted, is her mother's biggest problem at this stage.

Joyce is nearly 7 and severely deaf. She cannot hear high-pitched sounds at all, either with or without her hearing aid. She can hear some sounds with her hearing aid, including the human voice, if the person is close by and speaks fairly loudly. However, because she does not hear high-pitched sounds at all, the human voice is completely unintelligible to her.

She has been deaf since birth. The cause of the deafness is unknown. Her mother visited her doctor when Joyce was 14 months old because she was worried about Joyce's response to sound. He referred her to a specialist who diagnosed her as deaf. She was then about 18 months old.

She has a hearing aid which she wears continually. From 18 months she has had help from a peripatetic teacher who visited about once every two months. From the age of 3 years she has attended a day school for the deaf, 15 miles from her home.

Her mother communicates with her by gestures and the spoken word. Joyce is beginning to lip read and recognises about fifteen words. Joyce herself communicates by gesture, and occasionally drawing pictures of what she means. Her mother finds the biggest problem is explaining the whys and wherefores of various situations to Joyce.

Robin is 3 years old and moderately deaf. He usually hears someone calling to him if they shout, and he can understand simple phrases.

He was a rhesus baby and kept under observation for his first year because of this. Deafness was suspected at a year, though because of his erratic response to sound it was difficult to be sure. He had hearing tests at 18 months and 2 years, and at 2 the diagnosis of deafness was confirmed.

Robin has had a hearing aid for a year which he wears occasionally, and he has had two visits from a peripatetic teacher.

Although he makes a lot of sounds, he can only say three or four words and he himself communicates by gesture. His future schooling is uncertain.

Gillian is 6 years old and moderately deaf. She can hear the spoken word with her aid, and she understands her immediate family and they understand her, but she is reluctant to engage in any conversation with strangers.

The cause of her deafness is unknown. Her mother first took her to the doctor when she was 15 months old because she was worried about her poor speech development. He thought the mother was worrying unduly. It was not until a year later, after several visits to him, when the mother broke down in the doctor's surgery, that he arranged a visit to a specialist. Gillian's hearing loss was eventually diagnosed when she was 3. She was fitted with a hearing aid and had regular visits from a peripatetic teacher, and has made good progress from then. She now attends a partially hearing unit 10 miles from her home.

Her mother sees the biggest problem at present as getting Gillian integrated into the outside world. She is a very shy child and clams up with adults. Since she has started school she has few friends as the children who live nearby attend the local school and have formed their own friendship groups. Efforts to get Gillian to join in with them have failed. She is an only child.

Rupert is 4½ and partially hearing. He hears quite a lot: a shout close by without his aid, and with his aid he can hear most of what is said to him. He now understands most of what is said to him by his family if they take the trouble to talk directly to him. He has difficulty understanding people he does not know very well. He enjoys nursery rhymes and songs sung loudly close by. He has quite a large vocabulary and always uses speech to communicate, but outsiders have to make an effort to understand him.

The cause of his deafness is unknown. At about 15 months his mother had begun to get worried about him because he seemed slow in starting to talk. She could not put her finger on exactly what the problem was but she felt he seemed different from her other two children. She said of him at this time, 'He sometimes seemed to hear, but he did not take any notice; you couldn't keep him occupied for very long, he'd be wandering off while you were talking.' At 2 he could say one or two words, but his mother still felt there was something wrong. She said, 'It wasn't so much the words, it was that he did not understand me, he was never with me really.' She took him to her doctor, who arranged for him to see a specialist, and he was diagnosed as deaf.

He has had a hearing aid, and visits from a peripatetic teacher since he was 2. He responds more and more to different sounds with training. It is hoped that he will be able to attend the local infants' school, with continuing support from his peripatetic teacher.

His mother feels she has no real problems with him at the moment. She compares the present to the time when he was 2 and presenting many behaviour problems, and she did not know what was wrong. The present seems plain sailing compared with that time.

For certain parts of this study it seemed useful to ascertain whether the degree of hearing loss affected particular aspects of behaviour. In order to make statistical comparisons it was necessary to combine the categories further.

> i.e. more severe hearing loss
> categories 0 1 2 5 6   –   51% (62 children)
> less severe hearing loss
> categories 3 4 7 8   –   43% (52 children)
> (the remaining 7% (8 children) were not assessed)

In about half the cases, 52 per cent (63), the cause of the child's deafness was unknown. In the remainder the causes of deafness were as follows:

Genetic	2
Rubella	27
Meningitis	6
Premature birth	7
Rhesus baby	7
Measles	2
Measles and meningitis	1
Cerebral palsy	1
Bone formation of ears	1
Anoxia at birth	1
Toxaemia	1
Virus at seven weeks	1
Battered during birth	1
Damage to ear in accident	1

In the majority of the cases, 75 per cent (91), the child was known to have been deaf from birth. Eleven of the children were known to have become deaf after birth due to various illnesses or accidents, as shown in Table 1·5.

Age of Onset of Deafness				
birth	0–5 months	6–11 months	12–23 months	24+ months
Number of cases 91 (75%)	5 (4%)	2 (2%)	3 (2%)	1 (1%)

Table 1.5   Age of onset of deafness in this sample

In the remaining twenty cases the age of onset of the deafness was unknown.

Fourteen per cent (17) of the children were multiply handicapped in that they had handicaps additional to the deafness. These were as follows:

Physically handicapped	6
Hole in heart and other heart disorders	3
Mentally handicapped	2
Blind, and heart disorder	2
Cataract	1
Spina bifida	1
Physically handicapped and heart disorder	1
Lazy eye	1

About two-thirds (68) of the children were free from handicaps and in good health. Deaf children, though, do have a tendency to suffer from colds and catarrh, and in thirty-eight cases the mothers felt their deaf child suffered more from colds than normal children. Sixteen of the children were said by their mothers to be sickly, in that they were often ill.

Intelligence tests had formed part of the assessment procedure for these deaf children in thirty-two cases. Seventeen of the children were found to be of above average intelligence, eleven of average intelligence and four of below average intelligence. This is not to imply that deaf children are generally above average in intelligence. It seemed that if a deaf child was of above average intelligence he was more likely to be assessed with an intelligence test, sometimes due to parental pressure on the authorities, though in other cases due to parental willingness (and necessary resources) to take their child farther afield for an assessment.

NOTES

1 H. Keller (1902), *The Story of My Life* (Doubleday, New York).
2 'Sunday and Monday in Silence', a Thames Television production, broadcast 29 May 1973.

3 A similar result to this was found in an American study where over
   half the mothers of pre-school deaf children said that communication
   was their greatest problem. See K. P. Meadow (1967), 'The effect of
   early manual communication on the deaf child's development', unpublished PhD dissertation (University of California, Berkeley); or for
   a shorter report of this study see H. S. Schlesinger and K. P. Meadow
   (1972), *Sound and Sign: Childhood Deafness and Mental Health* (University of California Press, Berkeley), Ch. 5.
4 This is discussed in detail in Chapter 6.
5 The numbers refer to the number of these questions in the guided
   interview schedule. See Appendix I.
6 Quotes are taken verbatim from the tapes. Names, and in a few cases
   other minor details, are changed to respect the confidentiality of these
   interviews.
7 Many deaf children who are not at school see a peripatetic teacher of
   the deaf regularly. He or she may visit them in their homes, or they
   may attend a central clinic.

Chapter 2

The Deaf Child
at Play

In order to get a perspective on the young deaf child, let our
initial focus be the deaf child at play. What does he enjoy doing?
What does he do when he is on his own? As an introduction to this
whole area, the mothers were asked about their child's favourite
activities. Although there is no directly comparable data on 4-year-
olds, the range of answers indicated a variety of activities similar
to those that one would expect of normal children. Certainly the
diversity of activities would make one very wary of talking about
the typical deaf child.

A small selection of the replies are given below.

1 Boy, 4 years, moderately deaf
 Riding around on his bicycle. He really loves that. He'd ride
 around all day if I'd let him.

2 Girl, 3 years, severely deaf
 Racing around outside. She likes to be able to run about and
 make a noise. It's real misery for her if she has to stay in,
 you know – and for me. We're both fed up by the end of the
 day.

3 Girl, 4 years, partially hearing
 She's crazed on drawing at the moment. She's got these felt
 pens, you know, and she sits and draws. She's really good at
 it, you know, really good pictures.

4 Boy, 5 years, profoundly deaf
 He likes anything . . . I don't know what he likes the best . . .
 Jigsaws . . . Yes, jigsaws I'd say were favourite. At the
 moment anyway.

5   Girl, 4 years, severely deaf
She likes baking, and helping with washing up, and peeling
potatoes and everything. She doesn't really help but she likes
to think she does.

6   Boy, 3 years, profoundly deaf
He likes doing what I'm doing really. Anything, washing up,
vac-ing. He's always there. He wants to join in, so I try and
find – you know, I try and make it so there's something he
can do. I give him a duster, something like that.

7   Girl, 6 years, severely deaf
Oh yes, she'll have a tea party with her dolls and this sort
of thing. She'll try to make them clothes. She likes dressing
them and undressing them and washing them. All those
things, I suppose, a little girl does like and certainly she does
enjoy that.

8   Girl, 6 years, moderately deaf
She likes to have all the cushions out of the chairs and she
likes to pretend she's swimming. It's a great thing in her life
going swimming. She likes to put cushions all over the floor
and pretend she's diving in. She'll even put her swimsuit on
if we'll let her. She brings her towel and everything and
pretends she's going swimming.

The favourite activities of the children were grouped under
headings: active, quiet, helping and pretend games; and each
favourite activity was put into the category which seemed to suit
it most. Of the above examples, 1 and 2 are examples of active
games, 3 and 4 quiet games, 5 and 6 helping, and 7 and 8 pretend
games. From this it seemed that 41 per cent (50) liked active games,
30 per cent (37) liked quiet games, 16 per cent (20) liked helping
and 11 per cent (13) liked pretend games. Two children could not
be put into any category; of one of them the mother said her child
liked doing anything and everything with just no favourite at all,
and the only favourite activity of the other child was getting under
his mother's feet.

It is, of course, clear that the categories are only approximate
ones. The 'quiet' category would probably include most of the
pretend games. The reason pretend games are considered separately
is that they seemed of especial interest with deaf children in that
they are generally thought to be related to a child's ability to use
his own language. In fact, some writers have considered that deaf
children do not play pretend games as much as hearing children
because of the lack of the necessary language.[1]

To look at this capacity for make-believe in more detail, mothers were asked whether their children played pretend games at all.

Q48: Does N ever pretend to do things, or play at doing grown-up things? (Prompt as necessary: play at making tea, play the part of a mother, or doctor, or something like that?) Does he/she ever play with dolls?
If yes: What sort of game?

A number of examples are given to demonstrate the diversity in such games.

Boy, 3 years, moderately deaf
He imagines he's got a football and pretends to throw it, if it's been on television.

Boy, 3 years, partially hearing
He'll put two pencils together and that's an aeroplane – that sort of thing.

Girl, 4 years, severely deaf
She goes shopping. This afternoon my friend came along, and she'd got her doll's pram and the little boy, he's as old as Lynn, he was pushing the pram, and she was holding his arm to go for a walk.

Girl, 3 years, moderately deaf
She pretends to drink tea out of cups of sand and soil. And she likes to play kettle boiling. She puts pots on mounds of soil, and pretends it boils.

Girl, 6 years, moderately deaf
One particular game she likes to play – with Daddy rather than me – is prize-giving. He was at the prize-giving at school last year. It was the first time she'd seen this – but she gets out a pile of books on the table. You know what she wants of course, and she comes and sits over here and her Daddy's sitting down having his meal perhaps. He calls out names – she comes up and curtsies and shakes hands and takes her prize away. He calls out various names of children that he knows from her school. She'll tell them to hurry up – this sort of thing. She likes this. She thinks this is great fun.

Boy, 3 years, severely deaf
Now when he drives a car, he drives a car. If you bring his dinner in, or his tea – it's a case of wait. And he's got to put the car out of gear, he's got to switch the engine off, he's got to put the

brake on, he's got to do everything. He will not take it until everything's done.

Girl, 4 years, severely deaf
No, she pretends a post office. She's always liked the post office. She pretends to stamp . . . Oh, and bus conductors, this is the dog's lead she has over her head for the tickets, she winds it round and gives you your change, she's very good at that. She's got that off.

Boy, 4 years, moderately deaf
He pretends a motorway. He has pile-ups – everything. It's the M1 all over the front room when he starts. Ambulances, police cars. Everything. It's imagination – he's never really seen it.

Boy, 6 years, severely deaf
Well, he pretends to smoke and he pretends to go to the shops, and he pretends he's going out for a drink. See if we have a drink in the evening we show him, you know Mummy and Daddy are having a drink and things like that, and so when he has a drink he gets dressed up in fancy clothes and things like that and sits and pretends to have a drink. The biggest one I think is going to the shops. I can't go to the shops – he brings me things and asks me what I want and I tell him what I want from the shops and he goes to fetch them. Sometimes I have to join in but it's —— [his sister] who is co-operative, that lets me out. He'll be the shop-keeper as well. He sets himself a shop up, he's got a little till and things like that, he does quite well really.

There is clearly a qualitative difference of the degree of fantasy involved in the various pretend games. Pretending a motorway crash, with ambulances and police cars, is much more sophisticated than putting two sticks together to make an aeroplane. Pushing a pram around is a less complicated game than setting up a shop with a till and being a shop-keeper. It is possible to make a distinction between simple fantasy games which are simple isolated pretences, pretending to pour a cup of tea, pretending to drive a car; and extended fantasy games where the situation is developed, e.g. pretending a tea party or pretending a motorway pile-up. In the first four examples given, only simple fantasy was involved, whereas the second five involved much more complex situations. It is, of course, necessary to establish who initiated the complexity, for in some cases, although deaf children were involved in complex games, other children made the running. For this classification, i.e. for a situation to be categorised as extended fantasy, the deaf child must be in some sense an initiator. The fifth example given is a case in point, where although the father was involved, the little girl was obviously active in devising the situation. Looking at pretend games in this way, the incidence of extended fantasy was 43 per cent (52), of simple fantasy was 39 per cent (47). Nineteen per cent (23) of the children did not play games involving fantasy at all. As one might expect, the incidence and quality of fantasy games became greater with age. In the group of deaf children of 5 years and over, 71 per cent (24) enjoyed extended fantasy games while only 6 per cent (2) played no fantasy games at all. The degree of hearing loss did not make any difference to the amount of fantasy.

Not all deaf children played pretend games, but then, of course, not all hearing children do. It would seem quite clear though, that language is not a handicap at this stage, and that quite complex pretend games are possible without it. It may well be that assertions of difficulty in make-believe have been based on observations of groups of deaf children, for it is quite likely that it is difficult to get a group pretend situation off the ground where all the participants are deaf. In the majority of examples of pretend games given by mothers during these interviews, the deaf children were playing on their own. In the other example, deaf children were either playing with their parents or with hearing brothers and sisters or friends. Certainly young deaf children do enjoy fantasy games, often of an extended and complex nature.

In some cases the fantasy activities of the deaf child seem to the mother to be too extreme.

> Boy, 4 years, partially hearing
> He must have got a terrific imagination because at one stage I wondered if he was all right, because in fact he does it now, his arms go in all directions, and he seems to be talking to himself, having a conversation, and I mentioned this to Miss —— [teacher of the deaf] and she said 'Oh,' she said 'He's got a terrific imagination, of course it's all right.' I just wondered if he was all right mentally but she said 'Of course, there isn't a more intelligent child, it's just his imagination,' but that does worry me I must admit.

Often the imagination of the child worries the mother most when the child is seen to be in a world of his own.

> Boy, 3 years, severely deaf
> Usually he's happy. He seems to be in his own little world, and he's always laughing and that.

Boy, 4 years, moderately deaf
If you tell him off sometimes, he won't look at you. He doesn't
cry. He just stands in the corner or walks off, that gets me you
know. It's as if he's in his own little world.

This world of their own may include fantasy playmates.

Girl, 6 years, severely deaf
Yes, yes she goes off you, she goes off everything. She's in a
world of her own and she's talking to them. People, animals,
who knows – sometimes if it's an animal you'll see her, often it's
a cat – after she's been cross with it, she'll pick it up, put it in her
arms and stroke it. Cats tend to come into it more than anything
because she's a particular affection for cats.

It is well known that many hearing children, at this age, have a
pretend friend or even pretend friends that they play with. Sometimes such friends become so much a part of their lives that an
extra place has to be laid at table for them, and some mothers
even find themselves in embarrassing situations on crowded buses
or the like, when a space has to be left for the friend.[2]
Two points of view can be taken on imaginary friends and deaf
children. A commonly held view is that because deaf children
have not language they will be unable to develop imaginary
friends.[3] The alternative viewpoint is that since deaf children are
cut off from other people because of their lack of language, they
will develop imaginary friends to compensate. Certainly there were
many reports from the mothers of these children, of such playmates.

Boy, 3 years, moderately deaf
I sometimes bang the table and tell him to sit still, and he'll talk
to his friend by the side of him and tell him.
Q: Is it only at the table?
Sometimes when he's playing with his dinky toys he'll tell some-
one – it's as if he's talking to a friend.

Girl, 4 years, moderately deaf
She has an imaginary pupil. She'll run in and somebody's pushed
her over, and then this imaginary friend comes in the door and
it's 'Smack him . . .'

Boy, 3 years, severely deaf
There's a little boy, Robert, at school and he's always talking
to a Robert at home. He gets blamed for several things. If he's
got a scratch on his face, Robert's done it, this sort of thing.

Girl, 5 years, profoundly deaf
Oh – she'll talk, she'll talk away, yes. She'll talk to them, she'll express what she's doing, she'll show them and it's quite weird. It's quite funny really if you watch her, and she'll look past you, and talk past you, she's talking to this friend.

Although there is not the same richness of detail that there is in the account of imaginary friends by normal children, because deaf children have not the same ability to communicate, deaf children clearly do have imaginary friends. Newson and Newson, in their study of normal 4-year-old children,[4] took a strict definition of imaginary friends, where the same friend had to recur from day to day, and the child must talk of them as if they were real. The first criterion was adopted with imaginary friends of deaf children. The second was more difficult because very, very few deaf children had the language necessary to talk about an imaginary friend with their mothers. Even when mothers talk of their children 'talking' to imaginary friends, they are generally meaning a sort of scribble-talk, a pretend talk. The criterion used here for imaginary friends was that they should exist from day to day, and have some sort of consistent identity, however this was determined. The incidence of imaginary friends is given in Table 2.1.

Age		Incidence	
2–3·5	years[a]	4/27	(15%)
3·6–4·11	years[a]	10/42	(24%)
5·0+	years[a]	15/34	(44%)
Total	sample[b]	29/122	(24%)

Table 2.1 Incidence of imaginary friends among deaf children
[a] Age excluding immigrant group.
[b] Total sample including under-2-year-olds and immigrants.

The incidence of imaginary friends among normal children of 4 years is 22 per cent.[5] Hence if we compare the deaf $3\frac{1}{2}$–5-year-old group with hearing 4-year-olds we see that the incidence of imaginary friends is very similar. However, whereas with normal children, imaginary friends tend to occur before the age of 4[6], with deaf children the incidence increases after the age of 4. Mothers generally took such fantasy play and imaginary friends very much for granted – it was seen as a phase through which children go.

The mothers' attitude to children's noisy games or dirty games varied – as it did among mothers of normal 4-year-olds. Deaf children can make a lot of noise, and because they cannot hear it themselves it can be a very unpleasant noise. For some mothers this is intolerable.

Boy, 4 years, moderately deaf
He shouts; it gets on your nerves, really. Screaming and that, I can't stand it.

Mothers were often advised by their teachers of the deaf that it was of value for a deaf child to make a noise.[7] Through doing so, he can become aware of sound, and in particular the sound of his own voice. The majority of mothers tried to allow the child some freedom to make a noise, while on the other hand respecting the needs of their family and themselves.

Girl, 6 years, severely deaf
She can make a lot of noise at the right time. I object to her making a lot of noise if I'm wanting to – to be quiet somewhere, though I don't mind her then making a noise somewhere else, as long as I can have my quiet time where I want to be.

Girl, 6 years, severely deaf
If she wants to make a noise she makes it. One thing you couldn't – shouldn't stop. If she makes impossible noises for a long, long, long, long time – sometimes when she's singing – oh it's like the cats on the roof, it's really high-pitched stuff sometimes, and quite frankly you can't stand it, it goes straight through your ears you know. You have to stop it then. I say to her 'Sh . . . it's too loud, can you be a bit quieter, just a little bit quieter?' and in the end it's hardly there at all – poor little thing and I feel a bit mean about stopping because really she's – should be allowed to use her voice. See again us hearing people can only stand so much of it or you're driven crazy. The other two have got homework, and you can't concentrate on higher mathematics with a row like that going on.

Mothers of deaf children imposed less restriction on making a mess than they did on making a noise. This was seen by them to be an inevitable happening with young children, and to be accepted as such.

Boy, 4 years, moderately deaf
(Q41. Do you let him make a mess playing with water, or paint, or earth, or flour?)
Oh no – I don't mind. It's something we used to do once upon a time, I always say.

Some mothers saw such activities as being valuable for the child – learning through play.

Boy, 4 years, moderately deaf
No, not really. They're sort of finding out what it is and all that, aren't they?

Overall, parents of these deaf children were continually stressing the importance of play for the children's general development. Many mothers spent a great deal of time playing with their deaf child.

Girl, 6 years, severely deaf
I expect to spend more time with her, doing things with her, than I would have done with a normal child – I do expect to spend a lot of time occupying her, for the simple reason that when you're standing in the kitchen, you're not five people, you cannot be in the dining-room or the conservatory helping one small child. You have to show her how to do things – set her off with embroidery or knitting where I do half a row and then I leave her to get on.

Boy, 3 years, severely deaf
Oh yes, yes. Well again it's not like a normal child. When you get a child that's handicapped you find that you let your handicapped child do far more, because otherwise – with a normal child if they were sitting by you, pestering you, you'd say 'Oh play by yourself,' but you've got to train yourself with a handicapped child.

Boy, 3 years, severely deaf
I expect to spend time with him, because I've got to, how can I say, 'I've got to keep helping his handicap along.' He does play with himself a lot, but then if he wants me I get down and play with him. I get him to look at my lips.

One mother was prepared to devote all her waking hours to her deaf child.

Boy, 3 years, partially hearing
I don't do anything in the daytime but play with him. It's in the evenings I do my washing, all the jobs – scrubbing the floors and polishing them, that's a bit hard with his assistance, so all that sort of thing I have to do at night. The only thing I do do in the daytime is his bedroom, well I can't do that at night, and preparing meals and washing up, and he helps me while I do that.

When asked whether they did join in with their child's games 91 per
cent (111) replied that they did. In order to make a comparison
between deaf children and normal children, the deaf 3½-5-year-old
group was compared with the normal 4-year-olds, as shown in
Table 2.2.

	Mother participates	Mother does not participate
Deaf 3·6–4·11 years	88% (37)	12% (5)
Normal 4-year-olds	66%	33%

Table 2.2 Mother participation in the play of 4-year-old hearing
and 4-year-old deaf children

This indicates that more mothers of deaf children participate in
their children's games than mothers of hearing children.[8]

Various alternative reasons as to why this should be so suggest
themselves. Firstly mothers may feel, from being with their own deaf
children, that deaf children do benefit from more attention. Moreover, their meetings with doctors and teachers may reiterate this
point for them. Alternatively it may be that deaf children demand
more attention. When the mothers were asked 'Does he ever come
clinging around your skirts and wanting to be babied a bit?', 34 per
cent (41) mothers replied this occurred often, 30 per cent (37) said
it occurred sometimes and 36 per cent (44) said their children did
not. When we compare deaf 3½-5-year-olds with hearing 4-year-olds
we find they are very similar in their attention demands (Table
2.3).

	Demands Attention		
	often	sometimes	never
Deaf 3·6–4·11 years	17% (7)	40% (17)	43% (18)
Hearing 4-year-olds	16%	47%	37%

Table 2.3 Demands for attention of deaf children 3½-5 years, and
hearing 4-year-olds

However, when we come to look at the mothers' response to these
attention demands we find a difference between mothers of deaf
children and mothers of hearing children. Thirty-eight per cent (16)
of mothers of deaf children of 3½-5 years invariably responded to
their demands for attention, whereas only 6 per cent of the mothers
of hearing 4-year-old children did so. The reasons they gave for

their response varied in emphasis but centred on the theme that as they could not explain about waiting, it was easier or fairer to respond. Some stressed the expediency aspect of this.

Boy, 4 years, moderately deaf
Well I just have to leave and pay attention to him, 'cause if I don't it's tap-tap-tap until I do like.

Boy, 3 years, severely deaf
Let's put it like this. If you're doing something, and he wants something, it's far quicker to see to him, than it is to say to him 'I'm doing something – you'll have to wait', or try to make him wait. If you see to him first, get him happy, then you've got your time to do whatever you want to do. But if you try to do what you want to do he will persist, and he will persist, and he will persist. And I don't blame him, not at all.

Boy, 3 years, moderately deaf
I usually do it for a quiet life.

For others it was necessary to respond, because they could not explain to their child to wait, and felt it unfair to leave him.

Boy, 2 years, profoundly deaf
He doesn't want me to do very much really. Well, let me think. You see he doesn't speak so he doesn't ask me to do things, and if he wants me to do anything he touches me or grunts, and he wants his shoe fastening or his train fixing together and I more or less just do it, I think his life is frustrating enough without having to keep waiting for me to help him.

Boy, 4 years, severely deaf
Well sometimes I can carry on, but I usually don't ignore him, I break off and see to him, otherwise I think they can tend to get a bit frustrated can't they.

Boy, 4 years, severely deaf
Well I've learnt to drop and do as he says. I sort of think to myself 'Well they can't understand that I'm busy, and I'd like to get on with it', and I mean how can I put it across to them that J don't want to do? So I've learnt myself. I know at first I used to ignore them, but Paul's got such a habit of 'Aah-aah-aah' until he gets your attention, and you do as he tells you.

Another mother explained that whereas you can usually respond to a hearing child by talking, and not necessarily stopping what you are doing, with a deaf child you do have to stop.

Boy, 5 years, moderately deaf
I would think they need quite a lot of attention because you can't
shout to them – What do they want? I mean normal children
will shout – 'Mummy, how do you do so-and-so?' but you just
can't with Andrew. He just hollers and I come and see what it
is and have to tell him how to do it. They do take up an awful
lot of your time. I'll tell you the most aggravating thing. It's
always 'Mummy, mummy, mummy' where normal children just
shout what they want. He doesn't you see. It's just 'Mummy'.
Every few minutes 'Mummy, mummy, mummy', and you've got
to go and find out what it is.

Thus, deafness does not seem to affect the play activities of the
child, but does make a difference to the role of the mother in the
child's play. Mothers participate more in their children's games,
and many, though not all, find themselves often having to stop
what they are doing to attend to their deaf child.

We now come on to consider the effect of deafness on the
child's play with other children. Does not being unable to hear
affect the sort of group activities that a child can join in? Do other
children understand the attempts to communicate made by the
deaf child? As communication seemed to be a critical issue, one
of the questions put to mothers of deaf children was 'Does he make
himself understood with other children all right?'

Often between brothers and sisters there seemed to be a special
relationship and communication was easy.

Girl, 4 years, profoundly deaf
(here Samantha is deaf, Nicola is the younger, hearing sister)
They play together most of the time, because Nicola knows what
Samantha means. She doesn't speak very much, but she can
tick-tack and Nicola can do all that, she knows what she means,
and they play hours together, sort of make-believe games – I
don't understand half the games they play.

Girl, 6 years, severely deaf
Yes they appear to understand each other. They understand each
other quite well.

Sometimes this understanding between siblings leads to the hearing
sibling acting as translator for the deaf child.

Girl, 4 years, profoundly deaf
If they can't understand they ask Nicola, and she tells them.
She understands better than we do. Samantha will come in and

she'll go like this (gesture) and I'll say 'I don't know what you mean' you know, and that's the most frustrating part about it, when I can't understand her. She gets frustrated and I do. And I say 'Nicola, what does she want?' and she'll say 'Oh, she wants a ball.' And I'm amazed I am. I think 'How does she know that?' My neighbours find that as well. When Samantha goes round the corner to my friends – she went round the other day and she was doing all this signing and they just couldn't understand what she meant, and they asked Nicola, and she said 'Oh – she went to Michelle's party on Saturday.' You know, just like that.

In general children outside the family did seem to understand the deaf child.

Boy, 4 years, moderately deaf
Yes well, there's a girl, she's about the same age as me, she's got a little girl about the same age as our Bobby, starting at this school at Derby, and she used to come on a Monday. She used to live next door to me Mum. And they used to play together. Now this is something we could never fathom out, they used to play together, and they used to talk to each other. And they knew what each other was saying. And we could never fathom that out. They had a whole language of their own.

Boy, 6 years, severely deaf
Some understand him, the ones who've got patience to stand and listen, but he does I think in the end win out with them. Some children make an effort – the children are really very good. You hear that children are cruel but I must say that with Colin children have been marvellous.

Boy, 4 years, moderately deaf
It's funny, other children seem to understand them. Ever so funny really 'cause they do, they call for them, and they'll play with them.

Boy, 3 years, moderately deaf
We understand him, the whole family, and adults do, but the problem never seems to crop up with children. They just accept that he understands, whether he does or not.

This last quote points to what might be the crux of the matter. For very young children play does not involve the exchange of ideas. In fact the social play of children at this age has been described as parallel play. A group of children may be playing together with the same toys, but rather than the play of each being dependent on the play of the others, they are playing separately. In the majority of cases deaf children did play with other children with no communication problems.

There were some cases where problems arose, but this happened almost exclusively with the older children in the sample.

Girl, 4 years, moderately deaf
This little boy came over with his sisters and they were playing – and there again Jane was very nice to him, and he tried to tell her something, or ask her something and I had to go in and help explain and then he said very frustrated 'Oh she can't talk properly' and he's only her age, and that hurt me because he's so advanced for his age coming from him – so true.

Where the lack of communication did create a problem was in situations where arguments arose. A deaf child might come in crying but not be able to explain the source of his upset. Parents often mentioned how difficult it was in such situations to assess blame.

Boy, 4 years, moderately deaf
I suppose in the first instance we tend to blame John which is not always right. We are possibly aware of this – it's difficult really. At one stage I'd definitely say he'd be in the wrong and you'd be right blaming John – but this has changed now. He's not always the aggressor. Obviously as regards John, he's a bit limited in telling you what happened – and you know the other kids have obviously got the first opportunity to tell you what did happen. And this is it – so we obviously tread a bit carefully.

It may be for this reason that parents of deaf children are less likely to encourage aggression than parents of hearing children, as was indicated by their answer to the question 'Do you ever encourage N to hit another child back?' (Table 2.4).

	Yes	Special circumstances	No	N.A.
Deaf sample	40% (49)	27% (33)	26% (32)	7% (8)
Deaf 3·6–4·11 years	50% (21)	38% (16)	12% (5)	—
Hearing 4-year-olds	61%	21%	18%	—

Table 2.4   The encouragement of aggression in hearing and deaf children

In cases where the child was encouraged to be aggressive this was often to avoid being picked on.

Boy, 4 years, moderately deaf
A child like Richard, they tend to put on them a bit, you know. He will stick up for himself because his Dad's taught him to.

Boy, 3 years, moderately deaf
I would say if they hit you, you stand up for yourself. I don't think a child should be completely passive, but I would never ... if he hit another child first, then I would smack him, because I would . . . I wouldn't want him to be the aggressor. But if another child hit him, I wouldn't object to him standing up for himself, but I would definitely punish either of them if . . . I think spitefulness among children is very bad.

Some parents feel that not only do they have a problem in not being able to locate the difficulty in the arguments their deaf children get involved in, but that deaf children can be blamed for things they did not do.

Boy, 4 years, moderately deaf
One or two things have upset me a bit – what I've seen. It doesn't upset John, but he's got blamed if there's been children out playing and – well there was an instance a few days ago when the little girl fell off the form and I saw it happen and John wasn't anywhere near at the time, but Mother came out and John got blamed for it. It hurt me because he couldn't defend himself and say 'It wasn't me – I didn't do it.' There were about five children playing and John was the one that got sent away.

Girl, 5 years, profoundly deaf
Some of the kids, you know, take advantage of her. They think she can't come and tell me. She gets blamed for things she didn't do at all. They're inclined to blame her for things which go off, because she can't stand up for herself and tell you. That's the trouble with the children outside. She gets blamed for a lot she doesn't do.

In other situations, parents felt their deaf child was teased, and picked on because he had no redress.

Girl, 5 years, profoundly deaf
I think children can be very unkind. That's the only thing I've really noticed. Not adults but children seem to take advantage of her. They think they can do what they like with her, because

she can't come and tell me. They seem to keep poking her, or go out of their way to hit her.

In general, though, the deaf child does not seem to be submissive in games with other children. In answer to the question 'Does he stand up for himself, or does he let other children boss him around?' only 4 per cent of those children who did play with others were seen by their mothers as being submissive. Eighty-four per cent were seen as being able to look after themselves – as giving as good as they got. For the remaining 12 per cent it varied, depending who they played with, and the situation they were in.

Given, then, that understanding is not a major problem at this age, how much chance do deaf children get of playing with other children? The mothers were simply asked how much their child did play with other children (Table 2.5).

	Often (most days)	Sometimes	Never
Played with siblings[a]	67% (72)	28% (30)	5% (6)
Other children	57% (69)	32% (39)	11% (14)

Table 2.5 Frequency of play of deaf children with other children
  [a] Of the sample, 108 had brothers and sisters.

In order to compare this data with the data available for hearing children, we will compare the deaf $3\frac{1}{2}$–5-year-old group with normal 4-year-olds (Table 2.6).

	Often	Sometimes	Never
Play with siblings			
Deaf	63% (24)	26% (10)	11% (4)
Hearing	57%	24%	19%
Play with other children			
Deaf	57% (24)	36% (15)	7% (3)
Hearing	56%	37%	7%

Table 2.6 Comparison of frequency of play with other children, of deaf and hearing children

Clearly, then, there is very little difference, at this age, in the amount of play with other children of deaf and hearing children.

In many cases the deaf child was very popular and other children liked to play with him.

Boy, 4 years, severely deaf
No children seem to shun him at all, they've been quite good with him. He goes to quite a few birthday parties, he thinks that's lovely; once he knows them it's all right. He's shy at first, but he's really a good mixer.

Boy, 4 years, moderately deaf
Oh yes, they'll always play with him. They'll get him up. Even if he doesn't want to go like, they'll drag him in. I let him out on the road, they keep an eye on him.

Boy, 3 years, moderately deaf
(Q: How much does he play with other children?)
A tremendous amount. I never get rid of them. Can I play with Ray, can I play with Ray, can I play with Ray, all ages, I get them all here. I'm not exactly sure if it's Ray that's the great attraction, or Ray's toys. It's fifty-fifty.
(Q: Ray's got more toys?)
I don't say that, but he's got big things, a scooter, a car, a bike. He'll get sort of five friends and they'll all take turns swopping round, you see what I mean.

In this last quote, the mother describes how she made playing with her child more attractive by the provision of extra toys, a point which other mothers of deaf children may well feel is worth copying. Some mothers did make special efforts to get their child included in games with other children.

Boy, 4 years, severely deaf
I started asking children to come into the garden to play, and then they started asking my two to go back to their gardens, and for a little while they did seem a little bit afraid of Christopher because he wore this hearing aid in his ear, and they would point out the difference – Christopher wearing his hearing aid. A lot of them, of course, wanted to try it themselves, but I encouraged this and I explained to a lot of them why Christopher wore it, and they seemed to accept it.

Boy, 6 years, severely deaf
Oh, he loves to be with other children. I get him with other children as much as I can. These winter months it's difficult because Colin doesn't get home from school until twenty past four (Colin attends Partially Hearing Unit several miles away), and his school friends aren't round here though he does know all the boys around here because I make a point of having

them in for tea, sometimes he goes to their houses. He goes out
on his own, he goes and plays over the road on his own, he
goes off on his two-wheeler, he can ride that all right.

This last quote points to one of the problems that does arise as
the child gets older. Because he goes to a special school his school
friends are no longer local, and he no longer belongs to the local
group. For children of school-age, school usually is the dominating
force in their friendship patterns.

One mother felt that to make a special effort to integrate her
child with other children was to put the child at a disadvantage
rather than an advantage.

Girl, 6 years, severely deaf
We've only lived here a year, from last September. Well when
it came to about Easter Paula was going out to play on her own
and the other children were playing on their own and I – I was
worried at that time. Not particularly worried, because she was
obviously happy to watch them from her side of the road. They
would watch her and they just went on playing and she went
on playing. If they were playing with skipping ropes she would
come in and take her skipping rope out, but she wouldn't make
the slightest effort to go across and play with them. She'd sit
and watch them for a while and I thought this was awful and
I didn't know what to do about it. Everyone suggested why
didn't I ask someone over for tea, and why didn't I ask them
to come over and play with her, but the more I thought about
it – this might be all right as a solution, but Paula doesn't need
to be put at a disadvantage. I mean, I know her well enough to
know she really doesn't. So I just left it, rather reluctantly, and
eventually she just started playing with them, why in particular
I don't know. Sometimes she has children coming to call for
her, more often than not she says she's not going out, but so
do her brothers, I think this is because we're rather a close
family.

Though, in general, deaf children were included, there are some
examples of their being left out of games, though on many occasions
this was not deliberate.

Boy, 5 years, severely deaf
He isn't left out in the sense that they don't deliberately ignore
him, you do find that he's lost in the game, and unless someone
makes the effort to explain to him what it's all about, and to
show him the ropes he'll then go off and play by himself – quite

happily but . . . they don't really consciously ignore him, but
he can't cope with the game.

Boy, 6 years, severely deaf
Oh yes, he is left out sometimes in games. I don't stand and
watch him when he is playing, but when I look across the road
I sometimes see that he is being left behind – though he tends
just to tag on behind, he always sticks it out and forces his
way in.

Sometimes, the exclusion can come from the mother, rather
than the other children.

Girl, 5 years, profoundly deaf
I expect to spend a small amount. I amuse her to keep her in.
I don't like her to play out because I don't like the other children
tantalising her. There's always trouble. She gets angry and then
she starts hitting – and then the mothers come down, you know.

Girl, 3 years, severely deaf
There aren't other children round here that will play with her.
(Does she seem to want to play with them?)
Yes. She'll peep through the hedge. There're quite a few little
girls round here and she'll peep through the hedge at them, but
she won't cry or anything.
(Why won't they play?)
I don't know. They've never asked to play, and I've never let
them – they tend to make – not actual fun of her, but they're
sort of curious when she's got her hearing aid on, and they'll
say 'What's that?' and 'What's up with her?'

Occasionally the snub came from mothers of other children, and
not the children themselves. Mothers of deaf children seemed to
resent this rejection particularly, as it seemed to them to add
unnecessary problems for their children who already had enough
to cope with. One father, however, found such situations understandable.

Boy, 3 years, severely deaf
Mother: Only once I found that, when we were at the seaside,
and he was on the beach, and he'd got his aid on, and this lady
said 'Come away from him' and I got quite cross actually. And
I just turned round and said 'He hasn't got a disease' you know,
I was quite nasty I think. It really annoyed me to think he was
suffering because he was deaf, but that's the only time it's
happened.

Father: She wasn't necessarily snubbing him because he was deaf. I mean if Richard (his brother) went to a child on the beach who was a handicapped child, you'd have a tendency to say 'Come away boy' not because I don't want him to play with him, but because I'd be frightened that he'd hurt the child.[9]

Mothers were asked whether their children were left out of games or not (Table 2.7).

	Not left out	Left out
Total sample	64% (78)	36% (44)
2·0–3·5 years	67% (18)	33% (9)
3·6–4·11 years	71% (30)	29% (12)
5·0+ years	59% (20)	41% (14)

Table 2.7 The extent to which deaf children are left out of games

There does seem to be a tendency for deaf children to be more likely to be left out of games as they get older, particularly when they get over the age of 5 years. This may be because the games children play become more complex and language and communication is more important after the age of 5. Alternatively it may be because at 5 years hearing children start school, and their friendship patterns become school based. The deaf child in all likelihood attends a school outside his home area. This fact was pointed out by the mother of one child, commenting on her child growing older.

Girl, 6 years, moderately deaf
(attends a school a few miles from her home)
They're very nice to her. They all accept her quite happily, particularly at school, they've been marvellous to her at school. It's been really touching. She's accepted just like any other child. She had five of the children from school to her birthday party last week, as well as the children from around here. I mean, they ask her to all their parties. She's never been left out of anything. We are beginning to notice though that they do grow out of her a little bit as they grow older. She's beginning to take up with the younger ones. This will happen as she gets older we think.

The degree of hearing loss did not seem to affect whether or not children were left out (Table 2.8).

	Not left out	Left out
More severe hearing loss	68% (42)	32% (20)
Less severe hearing loss	67% (35)	32% (17)

Table 2.8 Effect of degree of hearing loss on child being left out of games

It has been suggested by some writers that deaf children are restricted in the extent of their social play because their parents feel they will be put in danger by playing in the street. Ewing, in a widely read book about deaf children,[10] states:

> Deaf children are restricted in their freedom to mix with other children because parents are reluctant to expose them to the possible risks of playing in the street, the park or the playground.

He bases this on work by Kendall[11] which I quote in full as it is a clear statement of a widely held view.

> When the numbers of children at each age level who were allowed to play with other children outside their homes, in the street or in parks and other green spaces, are compared it will be seen that this extension of the environment occurs quite early in the pre-school period for the hearing child, but that it is not a feature of the experience of the young deaf child. The reason for this is to be found in the parents' very reasonable fear that a child who is deaf may be injured through his inability to hear oncoming traffic. In addition, communication difficulties prevent the remoter control of his activities through preliminary warnings ('don't go too far away') or the immediate control through shouting from a distance.

Clearly this did create a problem for some of the mothers interviewed.

Boy, 3 years, moderately deaf
When I have to do things like fastening him in, it hurts me that. I think 'Oh it's cruel' but you have to be cruel to be kind really. It's either that or have him knocked down. That is one of my major problems.

Boy, 4 years, severely deaf
(deaf boy is Christopher, Nicholas is his younger brother)

When we first knew that he was deaf I used to shut Nicholas and Christopher in the back so that they couldn't get out, because really I was afraid of the traffic – you know Christopher getting on to the road. And with him not being able to hear I was so sure he would get run over.

Girl, 3 years, profoundly deaf
Well perhaps when I've been cutting the grass at the front and she'll come out and she'll go over to next door's and point – can I go over and play there, and I'll say no, and she gets upset then.

Boy, 3 years, moderately deaf
What makes Shaun miserable is that he can't go out of the gate, he can't go out with the rest of them. That's his only problem.

Girl, 6 years, moderately deaf
She loves to be with other children. Quite often, before she gets out of the car, when she comes home she tells me who she wants to play with. This I think will become more of a difficulty now because – this being a very quiet little road most of the children are allowed to go out quite freely and I haven't yet overcome my nervousness at letting Carol go. I don't know what I'm going to do this summer. I know that I've got to let her go, but I can't quite bring myself to admit that she's ready for it. I don't think she is. I'm not happy about this at all. This is a point that my husband and I have been discussing quite a bit recently. This summer she's going to be lonely unless we let her out with the others. But you see the river's not very far away. She could go along there and it's a very steep drop. You see quite a lot of people have got gates from their gardens through into the park – she could just be gone. (Q: Do the other children look after her at all?) Some of them do, yes, but they're mostly her own age of course, the ones that play with her.

Boy, 3 years, moderately deaf
Well if I have time I go in the front with him and watch, but more or less I'm tied all day, I've got to carry on, and there's plenty of space in the yard to play, but he doesn't want to be on his own you see. It's the school holidays that's the worse. The problem will be in these holidays this year. I shall more or less have to spend my time in the front – or put Heather in charge of him, but that really isn't fair to her. He wants to be with the others you see.

In these last two examples the mother considered putting the responsibility for the deaf child on the other children, but rejected it.

Some mothers felt that letting their child out on the road was an area of concern, but nevertheless felt that keeping a child in all the time was a worse alternative.

Boy, 5 years, profoundly deaf
It's just this past month, when he's been playing I've allowed him to play on the pavement. I used to keep him confined to the gate, the yard; but now I can trust him to go out and not go on the road. I keep watching him, it worries me all the time he's out there, but I know I've got to make him – I mean I can't keep him pinned in the yard for the rest of his life.

In fact, when we look at the figures for allowing children out to play, we find only 40 per cent were allowed out, 60 per cent were not. Although whether or not to let the child out to play is a decision not taken lightly, clearly safety is not the only factor – the child's social life is considered. Considering the problems, a surprising number do go out to play in the streets.

NOTES

1   Heider and Heider (1941) reported in M. M. Lewis (1963), *Language Thought and Personality in Infancy and Childhood* (Harrap, London).
2   J. and E. Newson (1968), *Four Years Old in an Urban Community* (Allen & Unwin, London).
3   See Lewis, op. cit.
4   Newson and Newson, op. cit.
5   Newson and Newson, op. cit.
6   M. Svendsen (1934), 'Children's imaginary companions', *Archives of Neurology and Psychiatry*, Vol. 32.
7   Not all teachers of the deaf would feel that any noise was desirable; some would prefer that only acceptable noises should be encouraged and developed.
8   $\chi^2 = 7\cdot3\ n = 1\ p < \cdot01$.
9   General attitudes to the handicapped are discussed in more detail in Chapter 9.
10   A. W. G. Ewing (ed.) (1957), *Educational Guidance and the Deaf Child* (Manchester University Press).
11   D. C. Kendall (1953), 'The mental development of young deaf children', unpublished PLO thesis (University of Manchester).

Chapter 3

Day-to-Day Living

For most mothers of young children, part of the day is taken up with routine tasks of caring for them: arranging meals, getting them up, putting them to bed, clearing up after them. What is the day-to-day routine for the mother of a deaf child? In some ways it is very similar, as I shall show in this chapter.

The mothers were asked how much they tried to get their children to look after themselves as far as matters of dressing, undressing, clearing up toys, going to the toilet were concerned. They were also asked how they felt about getting children to do things for themselves. As Newson and Newson[1] found with hearing 4-year-old children, there were a whole range of views from an insistence that a child should do things for himself, to a feeling that children were only young once, and should be looked after. Some mothers felt that caring for young children in this way was part of their role.

Boy, 3 years, moderately deaf
I don't think children should do much for themselves at any age, but that's a personal opinion. I think you do quite enough when you're adult.

Boy, 4 years, profoundly deaf
I don't want to force him into grown-up ways while he's a baby. They're still babies, and they still want a bit of babifying I think.

Many parents took their lead from the child.

Girl, 3 years, severely deaf
If they show they want to do it, encourage them by all means, but don't force them to do it, I wouldn't say that.

Girl, 6 years, moderately deaf
I like to let her do the things for herself that she wants to do.
I don't like to interfere if she's wanting to do it herself. I don't
even like dressing her in the mornings, because I know she'd
like to do it herself if she was awake enough. One tends to sort
of butt in because – it's quicker, but I think you get far more
cooperation from them if you let them do the things they want
to, rather than making them do the things they're not very
happy about doing.

As with hearing 4-year-olds, some mothers did feel that their deaf
children should show some degree of independence.

Girl, 4 years, severely deaf
I think she should learn to do all she's capable of doing, just
to broaden her own – well it's discipline, you know, that's
necessary. I think she should.

Boy, 5 years, moderately deaf
He has to do a lot of things for himself, because I think that
does make them that little bit more independent, and I think
when they get older they benefit from it.

Some mothers, in talking about their children looking after themselves did bring in the deafness as a factor. In some ways getting
a deaf child to be independent was seen as counteracting the deafness.

Boy, 3 years, severely deaf
What can I say – I think I've been harder with Paul than I was
with Peter, because he's got to do as much for himself as
possible, and we don't know how he'll grow up so I've got to
make him as independent as possible.

Boy, 3 years, moderately deaf
You've got to lessen their handicap, haven't you really.

Girl, 4 years, severely deaf
I think really when they're like that they need to be a bit more
independent than probably children that can hear you know.

The same kind of point was made when mothers were talking
about their child's behaviour at mealtimes. Here again, some of
them expressed the view that the child should be better behaved
to compensate in some way for his deafness.

Boy, 3 years, severely deaf
I would like to have a rule about waiting until everybody's

finished but I can't reason with him to sit there long enough. Here again, this is probably because Gary's handicapped. I think as far as, in my own mind, as far as dress and manners I think this helps people . . . you know, what's the word I want . . . to accept Gary really. I think if they have bad habits at table . . . I try very hard at this sort of thing because I know what would be acceptable to me.

Overall, though, the expectancies of the mothers as to their child's behaviour at mealtimes did not differ between deaf and hearing children (Table 3.1).

	Mother minds about child's manners	Mother does not mind about child's manners
Total deaf children	56% (68)	44% (54)
Deaf 3·6–4·11 years	74% (31)	26% (11)
Hearing 4-year-olds	69%	31%

Table 3.1   Mothers' attitude to child's table manners

Some mothers, although they were concerned about their child's table manners, did find themselves in difficulty when they tried to explain to a child what was expected of him.

Girl, 4 years, moderately deaf
I think it's nice to see a young child with decent table manners. It's been one regret that she's never conformed to how I would expect her to be at her age, but see communication was so bad, when we could have been teaching her nice manners, we couldn't even begin to talk, to explain what we expected of her.

Girl, 4 years, profoundly deaf
Sometimes she eats with her mouth . . . We've had more sessions over that than . . . She eats with her mouth open. And there we sit, and I'm trying to tell her to eat with her mouth shut, and then she'll do it the other way. She thinks it's a game you know, but you can't really tell her, you've got to show her, and it's very difficult, you know. It's all visual you see. You've got to mime with her.

Boy, 4 years, moderately deaf
Well, with him being deaf, we've had a bit of a job to make him understand – but he'll probably understand as he gets a bit older.

Girl, 6 years, moderately deaf
It is a bit of a problem, but here again we're beginning to win. Lately we've been showing her – you know – that you eat with your mouth closed, and although she will occasionally, with a great twinkle in her eye, have a jolly good go at making as much noise as she possibly can, she will really make a real effort to eat quietly now. We sort of mimic her – in fun of course – I mean we don't make this serious. We mimic her and make a terrible noise and then sort of say 'No' and then show her the proper way. She giggles of course and is silly about it for a while, but gradually the point gets across.

In the literature on deaf children it has been suggested that deaf children make a lot of noise when they eat: chewing, sucking, swallowing. Writers have attributed this to an absence of auditory feedback for deaf children i.e. because they cannot hear the noise they make they cannot tell they are doing it. Some mothers did mention this.

Boy, 4 years, severely deaf
I know you can't always be on at them, but it's really repulsive. He sits there (eating noise). I mean the noise and the food churning round in his mouth and I try and say 'Shut your mouth' and it does improve him.

However, it was not a real problem. Only 17 per cent of the deaf children made any noise at all, and the majority of these would stop when asked. Only 2 per cent (3) mothers felt that their child made a noise which they could not get him to stop. It may, of course, be a problem with older children, particularly in schools for the deaf, where there cannot be constant monitoring of every child's noise, and there is not the normal hubbub of conversation to drown such eating noises.

When we consider toilet training, again there does not seem to be much difference between deaf and normal children in terms of the age at which the mother considered their child was toilet trained. Furthermore, the same number of hearing 4-year-olds wet the bed as did deaf 4-year-olds.

The area of day-to-day care which seemed to be a real problem was bedtime and sleep. Going to bed is an important part of the day for any child, as described by Newson and Newson[2]. For both deaf and hearing children there is often a routine and ritual associated with a happy bedtime.

Girl, 3 years, profoundly deaf
Well I take her upstairs to the bathroom, and she gets undressed

and then she puts her clothes in the dirty washing basket and then she puts the plug in the sink and turns the taps on. And then she gets a sponge and gives it to me and I put soap on it and give her a wash, and comb her hair. Then she'll go and get her nightie from her bed and put it on, and then she'll go to the toilet, and then she'll run into her bedroom, jump into bed, and lie there while I cover her up. Then she points to the curtains, to shut the curtains. Then I have to go and kiss her, and I lie there for a couple of seconds, give her a hug. Then I close the door and she goes to sleep within five or ten minutes.

Boy, 3 years, moderately deaf
Well we go from one room to the other taking off each garment. You know, and then it's bathtime – run upstairs, thump, thump, thump, jump on the bed, in the bath, then down for supper, then another five minutes round the room, you know. It's chaos actually. He won't go without his sister. At one time he would when he was a baby, but now they both have to go together.

Girl, 4 years, severely deaf
I put her pyjamas on, and then she lays down with her Daddy. She usually lays there for about three quarters of an hour. Usually we have a run round before bedtime. She torments her Daddy, pulls his hair, all sorts, but then we take her to bed and that's it.

Many parents of deaf children, however, talked about the difficulty of getting their child off to bed and to sleep.[3]

Girl, 5 years, profoundly deaf
We keep trying to get her back in. If she starts getting up my husband stops with her until she's gone off – to make sure she doesn't get out. Because she gets too excited, you can't seem to get her off at all.

Girl, 6 years, moderately deaf
The worst habit of all is that she rubs her head on her pillow in an effort, presumably, to get herself off to sleep. We do have quite a lot of sleep problems actually, but she's always flung her head from side to side like this on her pillow. So much so that when I was using cotton pillow slips for her she would go through one, and she did rub her hair away, though it's much better now. We had a long spell without this – when she first started school she slept much better and I thought we'd overcome this, but she's gone back to it again now and we've gone back to having the sleep problems.

c

Some parents feel their difficulty is that they cannot establish a bedtime routine such as they would with hearing children.

Girl, 4 years, moderately deaf
When she gets into bed, we used to have to sit with her, but I say, 'No, I'll come and see you again in one minute,' and have to have a kiss and a cuddle. You see, if I could read her a little story, if we could get into that habit, but we can't, so I just sit with her, and if there's anything she wants to tell me, she'll have a little chat when she's laying down. Then I say 'Now don't get out, I'll come back and see you in one minute.' Well all being well we don't you see. That one minute, she's laying there waiting for it to come and she drops off.

Many find it easiest and best to let the child decide for himself when he wants to go to sleep.

Boy, 5 years, severely deaf
Now with the girls they went to bed at a stated time but here again you can't get through to him that it is bedtime. So I would rather him have another quarter of an hour boisterous playing, you know, to tire him out, than I would to just have him crying.

Boy, 3 years, moderately deaf
When Ray decides he wants to go to sleep he goes like that (snaps fingers) and there is no point in sitting with him awake asking him to go to sleep an hour and a half before he's ready to go. It's just a waste. I'm worn out trying to get Ray to go to sleep so it's a waste of effort.

Often the answer was just to go and sit with the child until he fell asleep.

Girl, 6 years, severely deaf
Well sometimes I go and sit with her for a little while. Normally all it would require I think is probably – well if she was well, and if it really was that she was just bothered about being on her own, it would just involve me sitting on the end of her bed, and I'd take my own book I wouldn't read to her at that time. I wouldn't make a game of it, I wouldn't even – put myself in the position of looking at her particularly to involve her with me, because that would keep her awake. But I'd be there, I'd read my own book or do some sewing or I'd knit. If she was frightened I'd be there. On occasions that has happened and she's just gone to sleep.

For many parents sitting with the child until he fell asleep was a regular routine.

Boy, 3 years, moderately deaf
I lay with him when he goes to bed, till he goes to sleep like.

Boy, 5 years, moderately deaf
We have to stop with him until he drops off. That's his one fear, being upstairs on his own.

Boy, 5 years, moderately deaf
He's afraid of going up to bed on his own. This is the one big problem with Wayne. He's always been a bit funny to get to bed. He's cried and cried when he's been left, and then when his deafness started he used to scream blue murder. I couldn't . . . his brother did this, but he didn't like being on his own, but I mastered him, made him stick it out, but I'm afraid with Wayne I was frightened of his nerves, you know, that I'm afraid I stop with him until he's gone to sleep. I lay down and pretend I'm going to sleep or else I wander around the bedroom. I'm just hoping that one of these nights he'll say he's a big boy and he'll go off himself because this is how he's mastered all his other things.

Boy, 3 years, partially hearing
Well, they usually go into bed between quarter to six and quarter past – and then they sit and read until I've tidied the supper things away and washed the pots, and then I go and read to them, I read them a story. Then they say their prayers which is something we're just getting round to doing. I lay him down and then I read a story to them, and then I usually read my book. I sit in there and read my book until they've both gone to sleep.

Sometimes it was not a simple matter of sitting for a few minutes until the child dropped off – the minutes could turn into hours.

Girl, 4 years, profoundly deaf
I stayed with her and held her hand because when we first moved here Samantha was one. I had a terrible time. I used to sit there, I was expecting Nicola, I used to sit there upstairs from seven o'clock at night and I used to hold her hand, and it used to be ten o'clock when I came down. You know, it got me so . . . she used to cry, we didn't know she was deaf then – I don't know what it was, whether it was the change of house, the wallpaper on the walls – I don't know what it was.

In some cases mothers had given up the idea of sitting with the child and just waited until he dropped off of his own accord and then took him to bed.

Girl, 4 years, severely deaf
You just can't put her to bed. She's just got to drop off and you take her up in her own good time. She can be up at six in the morning and she probably won't go to bed until ten at night. We don't know where she gets all the energy from.

Boy, 3 years, severely deaf
He goes to bed when he's tired. I never put him upstairs to bed on his own, unless he's asleep. He's never gone up awake, I get him ready and he'll go to sleep down here, either in my arms or on the settee, and then I take him up.

Boy, 5 years, severely deaf
Well he sleeps down here. He goes to sleep on the settee, or on Dad or my knee actually. He's not actually put in bed, to go to sleep. We like to know he's asleep before we put him up. But as I say it's usually before eight o'clock. And then when he's gone to sleep he's carried up to bed and that's it.

Yet another group of children went up to bed when their parents did.

Girl, 4 years, moderately deaf
Well that's one thing we can't solve so far, because she don't like going to bed early. We've tried it, she'll only go to bed when her Mum goes to bed. That might be about ten o'clock, eleven o'clock sometimes. She don't like going to bed early. If we put her to bed early she'll scream and come down.

Boy, 6 years, partially hearing
He goes when I go to bed, because if you take him to bed before, he'll go to sleep for an hour, and then he's wide awake again, and he'll want to come down and that's it, and in the night he'll often get up and walk around the house. He'll probably end up in somebody else's bed, and if he can't get in with somebody else he'll come down and bring his cover downstairs and end up on the settee.

Newson and Newson[4] defined an indulgent bedtime as being when the mother stayed with the child until he fell asleep. This could be in any variety of ways as has been illustrated above.

Either the mother sits with the child until he goes to sleep, or he falls asleep downstairs among the family and is only put to bed when he is asleep. In the whole group of deaf children, over a quarter – in fact 28 per cent (34) – had an indulgent bedtime. If we compare the deaf 3·6–4·11 years group with hearing 4-year-olds (Table 3.2) we find four times as many have an indulgent bedtime, a difference which is highly significant.[5] This would seem to be specifically related in some way to the handicap of deafness.

	Indulgent	Non-indulgent
Deaf 3·5–4·11 years	31% (13)	69% (29)
Hearing 4-year-olds	8%	92%

Table 3.2 Comparison of indulgent bedtimes for hearing and deaf 4-year-olds

Hewett,[6] in her study of 180 cerebral palsied children of 7 years and under, found 11 per cent had an indulgent bedtime, a figure which is very similar to 8 per cent of hearing 4-year-olds. Newson and Newson[7] suggests that indulgent bedtime for normal children often occurs where the child is the youngest, often after a large gap in the family, and indulgence at bedtime was a way of prolonging the babyhood of the last child. However, this did not apply to any of the deaf children who had an indulgent bedtime. Usually the indulgence at bedtime was a way of coping with what was to the parents a real problem of getting their child to sleep.

In the 4-year-old group bedtime tended to be later for deaf than for hearing children [8] (Table 3.3) although this difference was not statistically significant.

	Before 6.30	6.30–8.00	After 8.00
Deaf 3·6–4·11 years	7% (3)	62% (26)	31% (13)
Hearing 4-year-olds	10%	69%	21%

Table 3.3 Comparison of bedtime for hearing and deaf 4-year-olds

As well as difficulties in getting the child to sleep, there was also the problem of children waking up in the night. Twenty-five per cent (31) of the deaf children woke often and 17 per cent (21) woke sometimes. If we compare deaf and hearing 4-year-olds the difference is statistically significant[9] (Table 3.4).

	Often	Sometimes	Never
Deaf 3·6–4·11 years	26% (11)	14% (6)	59% (25)
Hearing 4-year-olds	7%	14%	80%

Table 3.4   Comparison of frequency of waking in the night for hearing and deaf 4-year-olds

Mothers described the problems that children waking in the night could cause.

Boy, 3 years, partially hearing
During the night, about three o'clock he'll come into our bed, he has done from . . . When he was a newborn baby we couldn't get no sleep with him and the doctor said to us 'Fetch him into bed, and if you lay on him he'll soon let you know', you know since then we've tried to get him out of bed but every night he comes in about three or four o'clock in the morning.

Girl, 4 years, profoundly deaf
She used to wake and scream every night. It used to drive us insane. Every single night she never slept through the whole night for months and months and months. It went on until she was four. Fear, insecurity, I don't know. We didn't know – we didn't know what we were doing for the first three years.

The mothers put forward a variety of suggestions as to why their deaf children did wake up more than their hearing contemporaries. One of the most common was the idea that it was not that the deaf child did in fact wake more often, but that he was more likely to disturb his parents when he did wake up. Because it would be dark, and because he would not be able to hear anything, he would be very cut off, and then need to waken his parents for reassurance.

	Dark	Other	None
2·0–3·5 years	11% (3)	37% (10)	56% (15)
3·6–4·11 years	17% (7)	59% (25)	29% (12)
5·0+ years	24% (8)	59% (20)	24% (8)

Table 3.5   The fears of deaf children by age[a]

[a] The percentages total more than 100 per cent as some children were afraid of the dark and other things

Boy, 4 years, severely deaf
He's very afraid of the dark. I don't know why – I'm only assuming . . . right from him being a very tiny little boy, when he was in his cot he was always afraid of the dark, so I bought a tiny little light – it only has a tiny bicycle bulb in it, but that's quite sufficient. I think that probably with him being deaf, if he wakes up in the night, especially in the winter time, and everywhere is dark, he can't see anyone and he can't hear anyone. I think this is what may cause his fear. He's had it as long as I can remember. He used to wake up screaming. I used to dash out of bed and put the landing light on – as soon as he saw the light, he didn't have to see me, he was all right, just that little bit of reassurance so that he could see where he was.

Boy. 6 years, partially hearing
He is frightened of the dark – you see we have a slot meter and one night he was fast asleep and the light went out and he was awake immediately. I think it might be with the deafness, because have you ever thought when you close your eyes you can hear, but him, when he closes his eyes, there's nothing. Well I wouldn't ever deprive him of a light – I know the girls never had a light, but I wouldn't do it to him. I mean no two children are alike anyway.

Boy, 3 years, moderately deaf
In the dark he can't see where he is. He's not frightened of the dark, I mean put him outside now and he won't be frightened. When he wakes up and it's pitch black he can't hear nothing and he can't see nothing and he starts to wonder.

Boy, 3 years, partially hearing
On one particular occasion, it was during the electricity strike wasn't it, you remember the lights went out at seven o'clock one morning, and he absolutely screamed the place down.

A related fear to this was the fear of some deaf children of being on their own.

Girl, 5 years, severely deaf
I think they probably feel lonely. They're in a world of their own in the daytime, and at night-time it must be awfully quiet because they haven't got their hearing aids on to hear.

Boy, 5 years, severely deaf
Up until he was two he was very difficult. Well in the end I put

Andrew (his brother) in with him – I realised he just wanted company. That really helped Darren. We had this for a long time that, even as a small baby, if Andrew had gone to sleep Darren had to wake him up and see that he was awake. And we also had it where Darren would get out of his own bed and fall asleep under Andrew's cot, night after night. And we'd have to pick him up and put him back into bed.

Boy, 3 years, partially hearing
We often think he wakes up and feels very insecure and lonely, if it is dark with the lights out, and this is one of the reasons we've left him in with his sister. We moved him out while we decorated the little room, and he seemed happier, so we left him there.

Sometimes the fear was tied with dreams, fear of monsters or the like.

Girl, 6 years, severely deaf
We had a spell of dreams where there was a great big animal used to come through the wall, and there'd be a second one. This was after they'd seen Dr Who on the television, and she was terrified, and every time she got into her bed, at the bottom of her bed which was next to the wall – it was a great big room which faced south – Pauline (her sister) and Helen shared it, and the wall would open – there was this invisible door in the wall. Well, all right – we had to play that one out too. We stuck a bit of paper on where she told me that the door was, and made a door handle, and then we opened the door and we looked inside – she was absolutely rigid with fear when I was doing all this – and then I whistled and called like you do to animals, and I patted them as they came out, one-by-one, and then they sat down with us, and we had to move Pauline's bed out because they were so big that there wasn't room you see. And in the end Helen was helping me to move the bed so that there was room for all these big animals to sit around and then we all shook hands and then they all went back through the door. We did this several times, and eventually one day they said good-bye, they said they were very sorry, they were crying, because they couldn't come back any more, because they were afraid that they'd had to go a long way away to see some more boys and girls. And that was the end of it. So we closed the door and took the door knob off, she took the door knob off herself, and that was the end of it.

This was of course the fear of a girl who could communicate. In view of the amount of fear of the dark which is expressed by some deaf children, it may well be that other deaf children do experience similar worries and anxieties which they just cannot communicate. It can be difficult to work out exactly what the deaf child is frightened of.

Girl, 3 years, moderately deaf
We used to have a lot of trouble. At the time she only slept about four hours a night, when she was between two and three. She just would not stay in bed. She'd do anything rather than go to bed. At one time we did have medicine to make her sleep, but you could give her double the dose and it didn't make her go to sleep. It was just when she was asleep it made her stay asleep, for two or three hours longer. But nothing made her go to sleep. We used to put her to bed at eight and at eleven she'd still be running up and down the stairs, and she'd be up at six the next morning . . . I used to sit and hold her hand all evening long, and the minute you pulled your hand away she'd sit up in bed . . . Well she must have been frightened of something. It was a big room, it had all the toys, there were plenty of things for her to play with. She always shared with her sister – she doesn't like being in a room on her own. And really don't . . . I never did put my hand on the trouble, I never did find out what it was – and the more she was in the open the less she seemed to sleep. It worked exactly the opposite to what it should really. I couldn't tire her out – we were tired before she was, and that's going all day long, and she would not sit, she wouldn't sit for even five minutes, she must be on the go. She was tired, but she just wouldn't give in. She held out as long as she possibly could, and many a morning I used to wake up on the floor. I slept the night, what of it was left, on the floor.

Boy, 5 years, moderately deaf
He's nervous . . . well I don't know whether it's nervous, but he just won't let me come out when he's going to bed at night. He was all right until he was eighteen months old, and then, he was in bed one night and he just howled. And I ran up for him, and we couldn't get him back up again. We were three whole weeks, with my neighbour who thought the world of him, we were three whole weeks, my husband, my neighbour and myself and we just could not get him upstairs. We found out afterwards, the light from the curtains, we had a road coming down opposite us, and car lights came down, and we think lights came through

the chink in the curtains, and it really did frighten him, and after that I used to stop with him while he went to sleep, and now I just can't break him of it.

Another reason for the deaf child waking up was given by parents who felt that deaf children did not need as much sleep as hearing children. As one mother put it, about her 4-year-old, profoundly deaf son

When you're hearing things all the time it tends to tire you, doesn't it? You know what I mean. In my opinion it's that makes you tired. With Martin there's none of that. He's in a world on his own isn't he? Martin is.

Boy, 3 years, moderately deaf
If I force Ray to go to bed at seven o'clock he will be awake most of the night. He doesn't need as much sleep as other children. He's never needed a lot of sleep. It's not that he's bad, he just wants to play.

Girl, 4 years, severely deaf
Somebody said their brain doesn't tire so much because she can't hear, but whether that's true I don't know.

In her study of blind children, Wood[10] found mothers expressing the same feeling: that due to their handicap the children did not seem to need as much sleep as normal children. She says 'The main source of the difficulty seemed to arise from the child not requiring as much sleep as his parents thought he "should" have.' Altogether 25 children were thought to need less sleep than most other children of their age; 23 'about the same amount', and 11 more sleep than other children. (It often happened that it was the more intelligent children who needed less sleep, and the additionals[11] who needed more). The conclusion reached by several mothers was that as the children could not release as much energy as other children by rushing about the house and yard, they could not become tired enough to welcome sleep. Although they would become 'mentally' tired and 'crotchety', after fairly short period of rest their parents would often find them playing in the middle of the night (even if they did not demand attention).

Other parents suggested more complex reasons than the simple lack of fatigue for their child's not sleeping.

Girl, 5 years, severely deaf
I think with her wakening in the night, she can't hear things if they're going to wake her up, so she has to wake up just in

case something is wakening her up. You know sometimes you have sort of light spasms of sleep. Well if there was a noise in one of your light spasms you'd wake up – I suppose unconsciously she knows that she wouldn't so she wakes up, wakes herself up to see what's going on.

Girl, 4, moderately deaf
Well I'm pretty convinced her not sleeping it's some sort of frustration, or some fear, and she can't explain it. It may be connected, it's one of those things you just don't know. It could be she's unsure of herself in some way, and always wants to feel that you are there, if she needs you. I don't know. I don't really understand how their little minds work.

Boy, 3 years, severely deaf
About six months ago we had quite a bad patch with him. He would waken up in the middle of the night and go wandering round downstairs, looking for cornflakes and this kind of thing and he would waken Ian or he'd come into our room. He was up a lot during the night and sometimes I never knew he'd been up. I'd just find things lying around in the morning. He'd take himself back to bed.

(Q: Do you think it was because of his deafness?) I think it wasn't normal. We couldn't quite get to the bottom of it really. I think it was like deprivation you know. I wasn't quite certain that he knew it was the middle of the night. It worried me a little bit. It was like sensory deprivation and he was going around trying to sort things out, or get things into place.

Girl, 6 years, moderately deaf
We do have problems over sleep. She has two distinct patterns. She'll either go up to bed, go immediately to sleep and then wake up about one in the morning and possibly be awake for as much as four hours. You don't always have to go to her, but she giggles and laughs, she sometimes shrieks laughing. You don't really know what she's doing sometimes and it's dark. She has no light, she doesn't have the light on. She laughs and giggles and throws herself around and gets up and goes to the toilet and goes back to bed. Either she does this, or she goes to bed at seven and plays around for hours. On these occasions she'll be contented as a rule, laughing and giggling – I don't know what she's laughing at. She laughs quite wildly sometimes. After so long she gets fed up – she calls and starts saying 'Carol downstairs'. Well, usually I take her a drink – try and settle her that

way but in the end sometimes we just have to bring her down-stairs. The extraordinary thing about this is – like last night we had to do this – about half past nine she cried, after having been awake all this time. I took her a drink and then she started to cry. I went up and said 'What's the matter, what are you crying for?' She said 'Carol cry, Carol cry.' I brought her down which we do very occasionally. You can bring her down, let her play around for ten minutes, take her back upstairs, and you can bet your bottom dollar in two minutes she's fast asleep – it's extra-ordinary this, and this has been so since she's been quite a small baby. It can't be reassurance she needs, she knows we're still here. She knows when she calls out she can hear us. She knows that she's not left alone, so what this is I just don't know. I mean if she happens to be like this and we've gone out and she's got a babysitter she's not worried. She doesn't mind, she'll play with the babysitter quite happily. Not a babysitter that she doesn't know of course, it's always somebody she knows. Some she knows better than others, but even if it's somebody she doesn't know terribly well she doesn't appear to worry.

The mothers' response to the situation of the child's waking was varied.

Girl, 4 years, moderately deaf
She has come down sometimes before we've come to bed and she's obviously had a bad dream, and I let her sit on my lap in here. Because she's usually dead beat, and her eyes are shutting already, but rather than make her go back into a semi-lit room, if she was frightened of something, I reassure her for a little while down here, and let her sit on my lap, and then she's gone again, and then after a few minutes I take her up and lay her down and she's already asleep.

Girl, 5 years, profoundly deaf
I don't think she is. Well if she wakes up in the night we have to have her in bed. She seems to have a lot of nightmares. I don't think she's frightened of the dark – I think it's more she's frightened of being on her own. She wakes up with a start as if she's been dreaming. She often wets so I think it's just that she's been dreaming. We find it's if she gets excited before she goes to bed so we try not to let her get excited.

Some mothers used a sleeping medicine, although often with reluctance.

Girl, 6 years, moderately deaf
I have got some stuff from the doctor to make her sleep and I
tend to use it now if we're having a babysitter, for instance,
because it is embarrassing. In fact we were getting to the stage
where we felt we couldn't go out and leave her. I mean we have
had babysitters here who've just been up and down all night.
We never go out anywhere to stay very late. I think it's just
literally she cannot get to sleep. Because she does try. You can
tell she's trying. I mean she'll say 'Carol's tired, Carol sleep.'
I think she can't relax. I imagine this is what it is, and she is a
hyperactive child. I think she does need the sleep, because usually
if she's had a bad night she tends to look pale and strained
the next day. This is why at last I've taken to giving her some
stuff occasionally to make her sleep, although I've resisted this
all along, because I don't like the idea of drugging her at all.
I don't want to give this to her, I usually – if for instance we've
had a run of bad nights, if we've had three bad nights, then the
fourth night I'll give her some stuff before I put her to bed. Or
of course if we've got a babysitter, I'd give her some stuff. You
see she does get so excited. This weekend for instance we've had
a friend staying with us and Carol thinks this is marvellous having
someone to give her attention. But she has got very overexcited
and she just hasn't been able to sleep.

Some parents take to desperate measures and use some sort of
restraint to keep the child in the bedroom. In nine cases (7%) this
occurred.

Boy, 3 years, severely deaf
He has a gate across the bedroom door to keep him in.

Boy, 2 years, severely deaf
. . . But we harness him in his cot, or we could never keep him
in. He would get out his cot time and time and time again, so
we use a harness, which he accepts now.

Boy, 5 years, severely deaf
I must explain that we lock him in at nights. It sounds very
cruel but it's for his own good because as a very small child
he would sleepwalk. So if he's wet it's because he's woken up
and not been able to wake anybody.

Boy, 2 years, severely deaf
He's in a bed but he has his pram harness on. This I don't
know the effect. Looking at it in theory I'd say it's very bad

and ought not to be, but in practice he's so active – it's for the sake of the sanity of the rest of us, rather than Francis. He would be out very early in the morning. He wakes up at about 5 a.m. some mornings.

This last quote demonstrates something which can be a very real problem for some parents: how to reconcile the needs of the family as a whole with the special needs of the deaf child. Often mothers find themselves doing things that they feel unhappy about in the long term, for the sake of a bit of peace in the immediate situation. For the mother below, where the whole family, mother, father, a deaf child and a small baby all had to sleep in the same room, the problem could seem insurmountable.

Boy, 4 years, profoundly deaf
We can't get him to bed. He only sleeps a couple of hours. He sleeps on a divan in our bedroom but he's only in it about two hours every night and then he's in with us, and that's it for the night. We nurse him, we always nurse him down here before we go up. You see we do have to get him to sleep before we take him because he wouldn't lay in bed. He'd make noises and scream and that, and he'd wake baby, you see. We've got the baby in with us as well. We're all in the same room you see, so Matthew's got to be asleep to go to bed. He's never been a child where you could go and put him upstairs, and come back down.

The whole business of the deaf child going to bed and getting to sleep does constitute a real problem. If a child is genuinely frightened how much reassurance can you give without spoiling him?

Girl, 5 years, profoundly deaf
We're lucky if we can get her up before nine. We do have a job with her. When she was quite small in fact we even got to locking the door, but I couldn't stand her banging on the door. I was too heartbroken. But the doctor told me I'd made a rod for my own back, giving in to her really, which I suppose I have. There's nothing worse than hearing a child banging on a door, and I thought 'Well I'm not going to have her frightened, thinking she's going to be locked in anywhere.' I would like her to go to bed earlier I really would. I mean it's no good for her. I've sat – my husband will tell you, I used to sit up there with her, and stroke her face, and talk to her, even though she couldn't hear me, and by the time I'd finished I used to be

nearly dropping off myself and Teresa would be wide awake. Because she just doesn't need the sleep. She doesn't need it. The doctors have said this – she just doesn't need the sleep, some children are like this.

Of course there are also practical problems in looking after deaf children. The practical problems are usually associated with potentially dangerous situations. If you know a child will not turn round when you call his name, will not hear you when you say 'No', forethought becomes much more necessary. The fire, the cooker, the power points, all become foci for danger.

Some parents could get attention by calling. Parents of more severely deaf children would clap or bang on the floor.

Boy, 4 years, partially hearing
I find that if I clap my hands, that's the quickest reaction. I've always done it and he realises . . . well at first, you see, I couldn't get his attention until I clapped a couple of times, and it would bring him round. Now, when I clap my hands, he knows that it's something immediate, you know, he's got to be.

Girl, 4 years, severely deaf
If she was going upstairs and I didn't want her to and I stamped on the bottom stair she would feel the vibrations and turn round and I could beckon her back, but if she's not looking – not really.

One mother had a most ingenious method. She kept a basket of small soft balls at strategic points, and threw them as necessary at her very active 2½-year-old boy. The gentle thud caused him to turn to his mother. It was difficult to see how this mother could have managed without such a system. During a two-and-a-quarter-hour interview she threw at least a dozen balls, all with good cause and all effectively.

For many mothers getting attention was a very real problem.

Boy, 5 years, moderately deaf
I suppose that's the hardest thing really, not now, but before. Because you couldn't get to him. I'd see him go to touch a hot saucepan and you'd shout but he wouldn't hear you – you'd got to run to him and a shout would have stopped him. He was difficult.

Because they could not call their child back from dangerous situations, many mothers went to great pains to teach children which things could be hot. Some mothers did this by going round indicating possible sources of danger.

Girl, 4 years, moderately deaf
Initially when she was very young and she went to touch the oven, or the electric kettle, I'd smack her hand and say 'Hurt', and she'd got a limited vocabulary, and everything I'd ever told her 'hurt' – she began to call them 'Hurts'. Even a little while back at school they fetched some scissors out for cutting, and she told the teacher they were 'Hurts'. And she came and said 'Did you used to tell her "hurt"?' and I said 'Yes anything I didn't want her to touch I said "hurt".' And she touched something one day, and it did hurt, and that's how she realised.

Girl, 4 years, severely deaf
By the time she was taking an interest in things like that, things that were dangerous, and could get them, she could lip read quite a bit. And I could tell her something was hot, and mime touching it and pulling my finger away quickly – that sort of thing.

Sometimes mothers constructed incidents themselves to show the child the source and consequences of the danger.

Boy, 3 years, severely deaf
Just let him feel, like the fire there, let him feel. He's never really gone for things like that.

Boy, 3 years, severely deaf
This is something he's accepted quite well, he doesn't go for them dangerous things now. Of course like all children he did when he was younger. I just used to say 'Mustn't touch', 'Burn', 'Naughty boy', you know. I used to take his hand and let him feel the heat and this has worked quite well. He did have an accident once, he managed to climb up into this chair – I was ironing at the back here, and he touched the iron. Of course we had great tears, but after that, now he's very cautious, he won't go near the iron any more.

As in this last example, mothers did find they could build on such an incident as getting burnt.

Boy, 3 years, moderately deaf
There again I've been there, and as he's gone towards the socket I've said 'Burny' and he knows when he goes near, and he says

'Burny'. One time he got burnt on the oven and I said 'Burny' and from then anything he went to touch I said 'Burny' and he learnt.

In one or two cases a fairly drastic demonstration was necessary.

Boy, 5 years, profoundly deaf
He used to keep turning the gas on, and I thought, how can I tell him, sort of show him that it will burn him, and that. I was at wits end you know because he was always doing it. Although I had a big fireguard and he couldn't get to the fire I was so frightened in case he put a pan over it or anything. So I . . . the kettle was hot, but not scalding hot, and I put his fingers on it to show that it was hot. I was in desperation knowing what to do. And he accepted it. He sort of jumped back and he looked at me as if to say 'You are wicked', but he accepted it and he never touched it again. And he learnt to say 'Hot'. He'd go '-o,-o', for 'hot' and whenever he'd go there and if he saw Pete (his father) touch the kettle he'd pull him back and say '-o'. When I told Pete he thought I was very cruel, but I'd got so I didn't know how to let him know. I thought as I'd sooner him have a little finger burn, than his whole body burnt. It's not worth it. (Q: What about power points?) I told him they was hot as well. I didn't know whether that was right. I went round showing him, and took him in the kitchen again and put his finger on the kettle, and told him they was hot as well, and he never touched them again.

Some children never seemed to learn whatever happened.

Boy, 4 years, moderately deaf
He won't learn. Well he's been burnt, and he's had his Dad's fingers with the electric drill, and he's been scalded with water. He tumbled into the washer.

When asked how they did explain to their children about dangerous situations they replied as shown in Table 3.6.
Of course, as well as the things in the home that have been mentioned, the road is another potential source of danger.

Girl, 4 years, severely deaf
One of the most difficult things for me is that I can't call her, this is one of the things that is always difficult with deafness. It strikes me most often when she runs to the road, or something like that, not that she would, but I can't get her attention. You have to be there to touch her.

Verbal	21% (25)
Gesture	7% (8)
Verbal and gesture	13% (16)
Punishment	28% (34)
Demonstration	9% (11)
Learnt alone	10% (12)
Does not know	11% (13)
Not applicable	2% (3)

Table 3.6   Mother's way of explaining danger to her deaf child

To what extent the road constitutes a major problem for deaf children compared with hearing children is difficult to ascertain.

Girl, 3 years, moderately deaf
Road sense is difficult. She knows she has to look, but the point is she doesn't always see – she knows what she's looking for, she can do it properly, but she's very lazy. She knows that if you're there, well you look, you see. She knows what she's got to look for, and she'll tell you when there's no cars, but not every time, and therefore I have to be so very, very careful. She's very quick. She's over before you can get to her.

Girl, 4 years, severely deaf
This morning we were crossing the street in town, and we'd both carefully looked and made sure there were no cars coming, and she was walking across the road holding the push-chair and we got just over halfway across and she saw a car coming on the side of the road that we were reaching; and she dashed back, and if I hadn't caught her arm she would have been under another car – she realised the danger from the car she could see although it wasn't anywhere near to her and so she dashed out of the way, but she didn't realise to look behind her before she ran.

Hearing clearly plays a part in road safety. The sounds of cars often provide the vital clue that it is necessary to look properly before venturing into the road. On the other hand, many people are aware of this and it is possible that parents take especial care to teach their deaf children road safety to compensate for it.

NOTES

1 J. and E. Newson (1968, *Four Years Old in an Urban Community* (Allen & Unwin, London).

2 J. and E. Newson, op. cit.
3 It is interesting to note that, while the sleeping problems described in the text occur with many deaf children, studies have shown that establishing a regular sleep cycle is a particular problem with children whose deafness is due to rubella.
4 J. and E. Newson, op. cit.
5 $\chi^2 = 20.67$ $n = 1$ $p < 0.001$
6 S. Hewett (1970), *The Family and the Handicapped Child* (Allen & Unwin, London).
7 J. and E. Newson, op. cit.
8 $\chi^2 = 2.37$ $n = 2$ not significant
9 $\chi^2 = 19.19$ $n = 2$ $p < 0.001$.
10 H. C. Wood (1970), 'Problems in the Development and Home Care of Pre-school Blind Children' (unpublished PhD thesis, University of Nottingham).
11 Children with handicaps in addition to their blindness.

Chapter 4

Discipline and Punishment

In all discussions of bringing up children, whether handicapped or not, the question of discipline and punishment rears its ugly head. Among parents in general there is a wide spectrum of views, ranging from the opinion that one must firmly enforce a given set of rules to a feeling that children should come to decide for themselves how they should behave. With parents of deaf children, too, both ends of this spectrum were represented.

Boy, 2 years, severely deaf
I've quite a different concept from many people, you know, not talking in terms of strict. I don't think the word applies. Children are children; they're developing human beings and you guide and assist their development, not for basic moral principles. I don't have a standard of table manners I expect him to reach, but I do hope to help him understand that he's not the only one at the table, and that he's got to take his place.

Girl, 4 years, profoundly deaf
You've just got to (smack deaf children). I mean you can't let them rule you. Once you let them get topside of you, you might as well pack up and go home. You've got to show them who's the boss, and you've got to stick it out to the end.

'I think he's got to be treated more like a normal child than a normal child'

Some parents were emphatic in the view that the best hope their child had of being integrated into normal adult society was to be treated as normally as possible. The same demands should be made of him, and the same punishment meted out to him if he fell short of what was expected.

Boy, 3 years, moderately deaf
I treated both mine the same. If they've done anything wrong and it's deserved a smack, that's it. That's all there is to it, he's got to be taught and they've both got to be treated the same. And the more I treat him normal, the better he is. He comes on better.

Boy, 3 years, moderately deaf
If I think they're getting it I smack them both. I don't pick on one or the other. I sort of sort them both out, grab one in each hand type of thing; because I don't think you should make any exception of him because he is deaf, because this would make him take advantage of it. I think he's got to be treated more as a normal child than a normal child.

Boy, 4 years, severely deaf
If it's a horrible noise I tell him so, because he can come out with horrible noises. I bring him up as a normal child, I don't treat him any different at all. Fair enough, if there was something other than deafness wrong with him you'd allow for these things, but just because they're deaf . . . Like my mother, she thinks because he's deaf, you should treat him different. She tries to. She thinks I'm hard on him, but I don't think so. I think it is hard. The more you drum things in that they should do at this early age, the better they'll get on when they're older, I think. Because they'll be on their own one day. I mean if you allow them to chuck things all over the floor, if you go out anywhere other people don't allow their children to do it.

However, for many parents this just did not seem feasible. It was simply not possible to treat their child as they would a normal hearing child. Having a deaf child puts parents in a different situation. Warnings and explanations cannot be given as easily, and a telling-off is not the same punishment if a child cannot hear. Above all, the common warning used with hearing children, 'If you do that I'll . . .', or perhaps more often 'If you do that again I'll . . .', cannot be used. A whole range of threats, warnings and punishments is removed.

'You've got to smack him to show him that it's wrong to do it'

Many parents found themselves in a dilemma in their attempts to treat their deaf child as they would a hearing child. From experience they found they had to be harder on a deaf child because often a smack was the only way to get a message across.

In fact there was a tendency for parents of deaf children to approve of smacking slightly more than parents of normal hearing children (Table 4.1).

As many mothers pointed out, with a deaf child, who cannot be told off, smacking can be the only way to get through.

Boy, 5 years, profoundly deaf
People said I was hard – I was cruel, but then you can't say to him 'That was naughty, if you do it again I'll smack you, or I'll take it off you.' You see, he wouldn't know what you meant, so you've got to smack to show him that it's wrong to do it.

Boy, 5 years, profoundly deaf
Well I think that's the only thing (a smack). It's sort of the way to tell them anything is wrong.

Girl, 2 years, moderately deaf
Well I don't really approve of smacking her all the while but it seems the only way that you can get over to her that it's wrong, you know.

Girl, 3 years, severely deaf
I think you have to smack, well not hard, but you have to smack a deaf child more. Well, there's no other way, there's no other way. Well there is no other way and anyone that says there is, well, I'd like to hear from him or her, because there is no other way. I'm not saying you've got to go and really, you know, bash the child about, but I think a smart tap, you know, I definitely think this.

Boy, 4 years, profoundly deaf
I think he gets more than what these other two do. I mean you can tell these not to do something, whereas you can't him.

	Approves of smacking	Disapproves of smacking
Deaf children	90% (110)	10% (12)
Deaf children 3·5–4·11 years	97% (41)	3% (1)
Normal 4-year-olds	83%	17%[a]

Table 4.1 Comparison of mothers of deaf and normal children— approval of smacking

[a] $\chi^2 = 5\cdot16$ $p < \cdot05$ The difference between deaf and normal 4-year-olds is significant at the 5 per cent level.

Girl, 3 years, severely deaf
Well, a normal child – no. I mean a telling off is quite enough. As for Diana, you can't tell her off, and there's certain things she's got to know that they're wrong. I think a slight tap on the hand or legs – she has to have.

'They don't understand and they think they're bad'

There is of course the alternative point of view that because a child is handicapped, he should suffer as little as possible, and be smacked less.

Girl, 4 years, severely deaf
I think because she's deaf it rests on you when you have done it (smacked her) you know. She is like that so you shouldn't. My kids feel you shouldn't do it to her, so she gets away with everything.

Other mothers suggested that one should smack less, for the very reason that some mothers suggested you should smack more – that the child could not understand what it is all about.

Boy, 4 years, moderately deaf
I wouldn't smack him more. I think you should smack them less, because they're not as capable as other children. I don't think you should smack them as often, because normally they don't understand and they think they're bad.

Girl, 4 years, severely deaf
I think if anything you would smack them less, because they have that much more difficulty in understanding what you're trying to teach them, and you have to take that into account.

Boy, 3 years, moderately deaf
I don't like to smack him, because he doesn't know what you're smacking him for sometimes.

And of course there were the one or two parents who just did not believe in smacking.

Boy, 5 years, moderately deaf
I don't think smacking children solves much. You get an upset child, you get an upset mother, and everybody else is upset. Quite honestly I don't believe in slapping children. To me it's bullyish, it's cowardly, you don't gain nothing by it.

Boy, 2 years, severely deaf
I don't believe in it. Certainly not at this stage.

In the group of mothers interviewed, although 10 per cent (12) disapproved of smacking in principle, only 7 per cent (9) claimed never to have hit their children.

'They don't understand what it's all about'

Of course there are many forms of punishment, other than smacking or verbal chastisement. Putting to bed, making the child sit still, ignoring the child – each of these forms of punishment was used by about one-third of parents.[1] A popular punishment with parents of a normal child was to deprive the child of sweets or television – a method employed by 69 per cent of parents of normal 4-year-old children. Only 14 per cent (17) of mothers of deaf children used this form of punishment, and only 5 per cent (2) of the mothers of deaf children in the 3·6–4·11-year-old age group. Presumably this is because such deprivations lose much of their point if you cannot explain to the child why they are taking place.

Boy, 5 years, severely deaf
No it's no use, you can deprive ordinary children as a punishment, but with deafness it's no use. They don't understand what it's about.

Major problems arose for parents who normally relied on verbal methods of control, parents who expected to explain to a child why he should or should not do various things, and felt they had somehow cheated the child by giving him categorical yes and no answers.

Girl, 4 years, moderately deaf
Well we could never get it through to her you see, that 'If you don't stop you'll go to bed in a minute,' so when she was younger and I told her 'You'll go to bed if you keep that up' and I followed my word through and put her to bed she'd scream hysterically in the bedroom. It wasn't fair to her. I'd have to go and get her out and think 'God, what am I going to do, I just can't explain to the child,' so bed as a punishment never meant anything.

Newson and Newson[2] found with normal 4-year-old children that middle-class parents are more likely to value verbal interaction and to use verbal means of control.[3]

One aspect of the difference appears in the characteristic attitude of middle class mothers . . . a preference for managing children as far as possible through the use of reasoning. Whether

the matter at issue is one of persuading or of preventing behaviour, the mother will try to give the child an explanation
rather than a bald command, and will be (theoretically at least)
prepared to countenance argument and to treat it with calmness
and further explanation.

Where, implicit in the parents' beliefs about the right and fair
way to behave towards one's children, there is a reliance upon
explanation, there is a clear strain on the parents.

A world without warnings and explanations can clearly be
frustrating for the children too. The warnings normally given to
children 'Bed in five minutes', 'If you do that again I'll take it
away,' cannot be given to many deaf children. Their world is one
of black and white, yes and no.

TEMPER TANTRUMS

With normal children, being thwarted in what they want to do
often leads to temper tantrums. This seems to happen with deaf
children also. These tantrums can involve lying on the floor, kicking, screaming, biting, etc.

Girl, 2 years, moderately deaf
Oh she just screams. She'll throw herself on the floor, bang her
head on the wall, take her shoes off, take her hearing aid out,
take her pants off, anything – you know. And she'll go and kick
the dog.

Boy, 4 years, severely deaf
He'll throw himself on the floor, his shoes will go up in the air.
I have this if I'm out and he wants a toy, you know. He'll pull
my hair, he did that quite often at one time, he had a spasm
of doing it. Once he gave me a nose-bleed, it was that hard.

Boy, 3 years, severely deaf
(Q: What does he do?)
He screams and holds his breath, and throws himself back in an
arch, you know. Which I immediately press him forward, because
it's not good for him.
(Q: How do you deal with it?)
I usually have to blow in his face to get him to get his breath
back.

Girl, 4 years, severely deaf
She still has a real temper. She stamps and if you try to pick her
up, she collapses her body and goes down on the floor in a

huddle and won't be picked up – she forces her weight into the ground somehow, she seems to be pulling herself down all the time, and if you get hold of her to pull her up she pulls away from you.

Girl, 3 years, severely deaf
Well she sort of goes all stiff and that's it. You can't do anything for her.

Girl, 4 years, moderately deaf
Lay on the floor, and kick and scream and shout and cry – every day mostly.

The word that was mentioned most often as indicating the root cause of the temper was 'frustration'.

Boy, 6 years, severely deaf
He did have really terrible tantrums but he doesn't have them now. Anything would start them off, but it usually boiled down to frustration. He'd just scream and rave and kick and shout, he never banged his head but generally go crackers.

Girl, 5 years, profoundly deaf
When she was tiny, every time we took her out she had a tantrum. It's when she can't make you understand what she wanted to do. You know if she wants something she can't make you understand she gets very angry then. Frustration, that's what it is.

As frustration seems to lie at the root of many tantrums, it is probably not surprising that the deaf have many more tantrums than their hearing counterparts (Table 4.2).

| | Frequency of Tantrums | | | |
	most days	once a week	sometimes	never
All deaf	54% (66)	13% (16)	20% (24)	12% (15)
Deaf 2·0–3·5 years	70% (19)	15% (4)	19% (5)	0% (0)
Deaf 3·6–4·11 years	55% (23)	17% (7)	17% (7)	12% (5)
Deaf 5·0+ years	35% (12)	12% (4)	35% (12)	17% (6)
Normal 4-year-olds		36%	32%	32%

Table 4.2 The frequency of temper tantrums among deaf children at various age levels, and normal children

At 3·6–4·11 years 72 per cent of deaf children had temper tantrums frequently, twice the number of temper tantrums of normal 4-year-children.[4] It will probably be a relief to parents of young deaf children to notice that the frequency of these tantrums decreases as the children get older. Seventy per cent of deaf 2·0–3·5-year-olds have tantrums most days compared with 35 per cent in the over-5-year-old group. No deaf children in the 2·0–3·5-year-group never have tantrums, whereas 17 per cent in the over-5-year-old group never do. Two-thirds of the parents saw their child's tantrums as being due to the frustration of not being able to communicate.

Frustration due to poor communication skills has been suggested by many workers in the field of deafness to lie at the root of these temper tantrums, and Ewing and Ewing suggest there is evidence that as the child develops linguistic skills the frequency of tantrums is less:

> Research has shown that for hearing impaired children there is a greater risk of temper tantrums than for unhandicapped children. Conversely there is evidence that deaf children have become less subject to temper tantrums as a result of good early training that has given them spoken language with a wide vocabulary.[5]

It would thus seem inevitable with the present educational policy which is committed to the development of spoken communication, and no other, with the later development of communication which that involves, that both parents and deaf children are to be involved in a period of frustration where the communication demands of the situation just cannot be met.

Many parents felt they could not get across the rights and wrongs of various situations, or give the warnings that are part and parcel of the day-to-day life of the hearing child. Only 32 per cent (39) of the mothers felt they could threaten punishment at all, and for the majority this was by showing the child the raised hand. Only 7 per cent (8) could explain enough to threaten verbally. It was even more difficult to promise rewards in advance. Only 5 per cent (6) mothers could get this idea across to their children.

The whole area of disciplining a deaf child is beset with difficulties. There is no normal way of behaving with a child who is not himself normal. Forms of discipline and control must be different because verbal means are restricted. On the one hand one has a child who has difficulties anyway because of his handicap, and for whom one does not wish to make life more difficult. Punishments out of the blue without initial warnings must seem just to add to the child's problems. One cannot have the same expectations as of a normal child in situations where it is difficult to explain to the deaf child what is expected of him. On the other hand most parents feel very wary of giving in to their child just because he is deaf. There is a further problem with deaf children. As has been pointed out in the previous chapter, there are some things which it is imperative to get across to the deaf child. Because they cannot be called back easily from dangerous situations, the hot stove, the busy road, their understanding of such dangers needs to be all the more certain. In some ways the expectations of behaviour of a deaf child can be greater than the demands made on a hearing child.

Girl, 5 years, severely deaf

If it's something really important she's got to know, whether it means smacking her or sending her to bed, it's something that you've got to do. I mean my mother thinks some of the things I do are cruel, but I've got to live with it, and if it meant giving her a good hiding or her getting hurt, I'd give her a good hiding any day. If she could hear, some things she'd never do so it's different.

Furthermore, many mothers of deaf children felt their main aim was to make their child acceptable in the world. Some mothers made the point that because their child was deaf he needed to be better behaved in other ways to make up for it.[6]

Girl, 6 years, severely deaf

I do think deaf children have to be better behaved than normal children. Therefore, I think they have to be nicer people. Now I've always had this at the back of my mind, though it doesn't always work out like this, for there are times when they're not. But at the back of my mind when I've been trying to do something, the thought has been there that they must be more polite than normal children. Strange noises they make, to put it realistically, have to be coupled with niceness and pleasantness and a nice smile, not tantrums and kicking the door.

Girl, 6 years, moderately deaf

We try very hard not to spoil her. I hate spoiled children. I think with a handicapped child they are sufficiently unacceptable anyway without you're adding to it by making them spoilt and badly behaved. We may even be a little bit hard on her in some respects because I feel that she's got to be acceptable to other people. I think this is very important – because I mean at the moment things she does are often appealing because she's small, but the older she gets the less appealing these little things will become, and I think these are the things you've got to watch. They've got to be pleasant, friendly children to be accepted by other people in spite of their handicap.

In fact, this idea that a deaf child has to be better behaved than his hearing counterparts is implied in much of the advice given to parents of deaf children. The following quotes from books and leaflets readily available to parents of deaf children indicate this.

In order that he may attain his greatest possible success in life [the deaf child] must be a little better than his hearing fellows. He needs to be more courteous, more considerate of others, more energetic, more ambitious and more efficient. He must be willing to work harder, to take more pains to do his work well, to be more alert in recognising needs and opportunities.[7]

The most effective discipline is firm, timely and consistent and is tempered with a thorough understanding of the child's problem. If anything, discipline should be stricter than for hearing children in the earlier years because a deaf child's limited vocabulary prevents a parent from reasoning with him. He must learn to obey if he is to fit in socially.[8]

Be firm with your deaf baby, though in a kindly happy way. Remember – deaf babies, deaf children and ultimately deaf adults have to live in a world of hearing people, and the more easily they fit in the happier their lives will be. *You can see the reason for this, can't you?* (author's italics)[9]

Clearly it is almost impossible to bring up a deaf child in the way that you would a hearing child. In such an already difficult situation the idea of an extra hurdle, i.e. that success and integration depend on the deaf child being better behaved than his hearing counterparts, seems a little unfair.

Mothers of deaf children did, in fact, give a lot of thought to trying to work out the best way to cope with their handicapped child.

Girl, 4 years, severely deaf
I always feel I'm wrong if I've smacked her, but I think otherwise we don't do too badly. I wonder sometimes if we give in a bit too much – not so much giving in to what she wants, but making it convenient for her to have what she wants – you know I sometimes think we do that a bit too much with her. I think we do it more than we would if she could hear.

Girl, 4 years, moderately deaf
No, I worry sometimes, whether I'm doing the right thing or . . .
See everyone used to say at first, when she was younger, that I
was too strict with her, too hard on her – she was only a child.
But there again, the only alternative I could see was to give in
to her and have a thoroughly spoilt child. I just handled her the
way I thought best, but unfortunately my temper isn't what it
should be – it leaves plenty to be desired. So I wonder if in the
heat of the moment, with my bad temper, I really do overdo
things.

Girl, 3 years, severely deaf
Well sometimes in the punishment line, you know, sometimes
I think, well I don't know . . . am I doing . . . I question my own
. . . well . . . I think well am I doing right. Not being quite sure
whether. I maintain you've got to be really firm, you've got to
tap deaf children to get over to them more. It's hard coping with
a deaf child, it's terribly hard coping with a deaf child particularly in discipline.

Boy, 4 years, severely deaf
Sometimes I wonder to myself whether I'm doing the right thing
or not. Sometimes I think to myself – should I have brought him
up differently because he is handicapped, did I ought to treat
him differently, did I ought to try to make it up to him in other
little ways, because he's deaf. At this stage it is a bit of a problem to know whether you are doing the right thing or not, I
suppose later on it will be proved to me whether I have done
the right thing or not.

'You're only human as well, aren't you?'

Many parents pointed out that the situation could not only be frustrating for the child, but could be frustrating for them too. Often
they behaved in ways that they later regretted through sheer frustration or overtiredness.

Boy, 3 years, moderately deaf
I probably do a lot that I don't really approve of. I've never
really smacked the others hard, I probably smack him more than
I've smacked them. And when he's frustrated I think you do
things that you'd never do normally, you know. You're probably
harder with him altogether. I find I shout a lot at him, which
I, we tried not to do, but if he's really naughty I shout at him

and say 'Go away, leave me alone', something like this. And you can see he changes straight away and gets upset . . . I think all parents of deaf children go through a stage, when they're very young you can't do anything and you're frustrated probably from that. I think it's a hangover from when they're very little.

Boy, 6 years, severely deaf
I find myself when I am screaming and raving. I mean I scream and rave – I get quite ashamed of myself over that but then I sort of say to myself well, if I didn't do that I think I'd go mental. If I didn't let go you see.

Boy, 3 years, moderately deaf
Oh yes, sometimes I think I've let him go a bit too far, or clouted him a bit hard. But on the other hand it takes so much out of you, you have to be really good not to . . . you're only human as well aren't you, d'you know what I mean? I think sometimes that, well, I shouldn't have done that because I've taken it out on him and it's something else that's niggled me, you know, but he takes it out of me sometimes, I suppose.

Girl, 5 years, severely deaf
Sometimes I think I smack her too much, and then it passes and the next time she gets a smack. Sometimes I feel guilty in myself because I moan at her. Really it boils down to that hearing aids upset me for the noise, especially if you're a bit under the weather it irritates you more than anything. There's nothing you can alter, you can't keep it clear all the time especially when they're playing. And if she's reading you see the book comes in front of it and then it starts whistling, and as I say if you are under the weather it does start to irritate you.

Boy, 4 years, partially hearing
I don't know really. We do disagree, but that's mostly because I'm overtired, and I haven't got the patience. It's mostly my fault, you know, if I'm overtired, I get a bit irritable.

Many mothers did try and take an objective view of the situation. Their general approach was that, bearing in mind the problems in the situation, they felt they did cope as best they could.

Girl, 6 years, moderately deaf
Well I wouldn't say I find myself doing things I don't approve of, but I often wonder if I'm doing the right thing. Well of course sometimes I've got cross and smacked her and then afterwards I've thought well that was stupid. There was no reason

why she shouldn't have been doing what she was doing necessarily – but then I think it's a question of how you're feeling at
the time. Sometimes I've thought well I wouldn't let her do that
and then I let her do it because she's not doing any harm. She
might have made a bit of a mess, but so what? Occasionally I've
felt self-critical on those grounds. On the whole I think we've got
a fairly reasonable pattern of dealing with her.

Girl, 6 years, severely deaf
You're never entirely happy with the way you handle any child,
are you? On the whole I don't see how you can be any different
from the person you are – how you would behave with a child.
The fact that that child is different and has to be treated at a
more slower pace with everything she does – she has the handicap of not hearing – to allow for this, and you yourself only act
in the way that you see it, the way you feel about it. You get
discouraged because you're not doing enough, that you're not
doing it well enough. But – when you inquire from other people,
sometimes other parents, and doctors, and clinics and hospitals,
wherever we've been – we've been to some peculiar places, and
we've met some of the most peculiar people who were supposed
to be very intelligent, incidentally, some of them – we've asked
questions of them but never got any answers that you felt
would apply, that would have a better effect than what you're
already doing. Because we've just – we've always tried to bring
her up the way we've brought the others up. Except for sound
communication I must accept that she's about two years old in
actual sound, but intelligent communication other than sound,
with relevant sounds that she makes is six to seven-year-old
behaviour. You can't get much nearer than that can you.

About half the mothers of deaf children (58 per cent, 59) were
critical about the way they were bringing up their children – a very

	Mothers' Self Rating			
	very strict	rather strict	rather easy	very easy
All deaf Deaf	9% (11)	39% (47)	38% (46)	15% (18)
3·5–4·11 years Normal	7% (3)	40% (17)	33% (14)	19% (8)
4-year-olds	3%	36%	51%	10%

Table 4.3 Mothers self ratings on strictness

similar figure to the self-criticism among mothers of normal children (54 per cent). However, when asked to rate themselves on how strict they were, there was a tendency for them to feel that they were more strict with their deaf children (Table 4.3).

NOTES

1 Sending to bed   30% (37)
   Sit still   31% (38)
   Ignore child   32% (39)
2 J. and E. Newson (1968), *Four Years Old in an Urban Community* (Allen & Unwin, London).
3 This point is reiterated in the work of Bernstein and his colleagues. See J. Cook-Gumperz (1973), *Social Control and Socialisation* (Routledge & Kegan Paul, London).
4 This difference is highly significant: $\chi^2 = 19 \cdot 27$ $p < \cdot 001$.
5 A. Ewing and E. C. Ewing (1971), *Hearing – Impaired Children Under Five* (Manchester University Press).
6 See above pp. 62–63.
7 John Tracey Clinic Correspondence Course, quoted in D. M. C. Dale (1967), *Deaf Children at Home and School* (University of London Press).
8 D. M. C. Dale, op. cit.
9 K. M. Williams (1972), *You Can Help Your Deaf Baby* (National College of Teachers of the Deaf).

D

Chapter 5

Learning to Communicate: Equipment

It is very clear from the preceding chapters that the basic problem of deaf children is not that they cannot hear, but that communication between themselves and others is difficult. Learning to communicate presents the deaf with increased problems. In these next two chapters we shall consider what help is available to the deaf child and his parents in developing an ability in the child to communicate.

The first and obvious type of help is a hearing aid. Most children have some hearing. A hearing aid can amplify what sounds they do hear.

Other equipment available is a speech trainer, similar to a body-worn aid in principle, but which has larger and more efficient earphones and microphone. It has the disadvantage that it is cumbersome and can only be used for as long as the child is prepared to stay in the same place, but it gives much better amplification of sound with less distortion. It is usually used for short periods and for more intensive work.

For virtually all deaf children a hearing aid is essential equipment. Most deaf children do have some hearing and a hearing aid can amplify what sounds they do hear. However, it must be made clear at the outset that even the very best hearing aid has its limitations. Many people expect a hearing aid to do for a hearing loss what spectacles do for defective vision. Spectacles make vision normal for the wearer.[1] A hearing aid does not restore its user to normal hearing. Firstly, it can only amplify what the person can hear – so if they hear low pitch sounds but not high pitch sounds they will continue to hear low pitch sound only, but this will be louder. Secondly, binaural hearing (hearing with two ears) allows us to select certain sounds to attend to. We hear our own name across a crowded room when in fact it was said no louder than any other name which is mentioned. A hearing aid cannot select in this way. A hearing aid in each ear is better, but does not necessarily allow such selection. Listening to a tape recording made in a crowded room will give some indication of what happens when every sound is picked up and none are filtered out. Thirdly, there is feedback between the amplifier and the microphone unless they are carefully adjusted. This means that the microphone picks up sounds going through the amplifier causing a whistle. (This is a vastly oversimplified explanation.)[2]

Despite such problems, the essential equipment for a deaf child is a hearing aid. As the recent report on the education of deaf children put it:[3]

Experience has shown clearly that in all but a few cases, other factors being equal, children deaf from birth or early infancy make better progress if they are fitted in babyhood with suitable hearing aids, prescribed by an otologist, and encouraged to wear the aids continuously and are trained to listen. Naturally, these measures will be helpful only if the aid is kept in good working order and is used in reasonably good acoustic conditions. Some children with severe hearing loss can be helped to discriminate speech and even those who hear relatively little amplified sound and cannot discriminate words may be helped to detect some of the rhythms and other patterns of normal speech and to gain clues to meaning which they would otherwise miss. Comprehension is greater when children combine the use of residual hearing and lip reading than when either of these methods are used alone.

If we can enumerate the points put forward in this paragraph:

(a) the child should be fitted in babyhood with an aid;
(b) the aid should be suitable;
(c) he should wear the aid continuously;
(d) he should be taught to listen;
(e) the aid should be kept in good working order;
(f) it should be used in reasonably good acoustic conditions;
(g) residual hearing and lip reading should be combined to give the best results.

All writers on the education of deaf children would be in accord upon these points, so perhaps we can take them one by one. (Points (d) (f) and (g) are dealt with in the section on peripatetic teachers).

(a) *The child should be fitted in babyhood with an aid.* The age at which the children in this sample first were supplied with aids is given in Table 5.1.

Age	Number of children
Less than 12 months	11 (9%)
13–18 months	26 (21%)
19–24 months	21 (17%)
25–36 months	39 (32%)
37 months and over	17 (14%)
No aid	8 (7%)

Table 5.1   Age at which children were supplied with hearing aids

However this does not show the whole picture as not all children are diagnosed in babyhood. A more realistic approach is to take the time from diagnosis to the supply of the aid. This is given in Table 5.2.

Time	Number of children
1 week or less	26% (30)
2–4 weeks	44% (50)
5–15 weeks	20% (23)
4–6 months	4% (5)
6 months or more	5% (6)

Table 5.2   Time from diagnosis to supply of aid

From this we see that over two-thirds of the children were supplied with a hearing aid within four weeks of being diagnosed for deafness. There is cause for concern in that 9 per cent of children had to wait four months or more for a hearing aid. A problem for the mothers is that they do not know what is a reasonable time to wait for an aid, or how important an aid is considered to be.

Girl, 3 years, moderately deaf
The person that did the moulds said 'This child could have had an aid a lot sooner.' I think that when they know that your child is deaf they should issue you with an aid while they're trying to find out how deaf, because that way right from the start she's getting benefit. If she doesn't need it then she's not lost anything. She could have had it four months earlier than she did.

Boy, 3 years, partially hearing
It was a lady doctor, and she said he could be helped with a

hearing aid. And I thought that would be immediate and it wasn't – not until he was two (one year later).

(Q: Do you remember what she actually said to you?) She said he was totally deaf, she thought he was worse actually, than – well I wouldn't say totally deaf, but she thought he was very seriously . . . She put me in touch with a peripatetic teacher that was here at that time, and that was all we knew.

As I say we knew very little about this problem, I mean even myself as a nurse – I've never met young children with this sort of problem, because we didn't get it at the hospitals. Had I known then what I know now, he would have had an aid straight away, because to me, even I can understand that he missed out at the wrong time, you know. Just at the time when he would be able to do the normal learning of speech he was missing out.

In fact one would wish to add to the proviso that the child should be fitted in babyhood with an aid, that the parents should be given advice about the use of the aid, and what they can expect from it. Unless a mother is forewarned she is very likely to expect the aid to restore the child to perfect hearing. One mother told how the aid for her little girl had come through the post. She did all her housework, put the little girl in her best dress, put in the aid in anticipation that her daughter would now be able to hear – but her daughter tore the aid out of her ear. She did not want to know. Another mother told a similar story.

Boy, 3 years, severely deaf
No, they just . . . see they fitted him up with it, and I asked them . . . I thought he could hear then you see. I said er . . . 'Can he hear?' and they said 'Oh we don't know,' and that was it you see. And I didn't know how I was supposed to tell, and I thought we'd be able to tell as soon as he'd got it in, we'd be able to tell whether he could hear or not, I expected this miraculous thing to happen but it didn't make any impression to start with. I expected to see his whole face light up – he could hear – but it didn't.

Clearly, to supply an aid is just not enough.
Even for those mothers who did not have high expectations, information on the use of the aid is necessary. How long should the child wear it? Should he wear it under or over his clothes? How often will the batteries need renewing? What does it mean when it whistles?[4] What number should the aid be set on?
Some parents had no help at all.

Boy, 3 years, moderately deaf
I wasn't even told how to put the ear pieces in. No, they just said 'Here's your hearing aid, switch it to whatever you think he needs, it's all yours.' That was the lot. We just sort of spent the evening experimenting on ourselves actually.

Boy, 5 years, moderately deaf
Well we didn't (get any advice) because we were just sent it by post. We just put it in. We didn't know what number to put it on so we just put it in and hoped for the best.

Girl, 3 years, severely deaf
They just stuck it on her and that was it. They didn't say anything about it.

Some parents had some advice, often a booklet, but where this advice was only about the maintenance of the aid, or obviously inadequate in other ways, I have described it as minimal advice.

Girl, 5 years, moderately deaf
They just gave me a book, you know, which just showed me the On and Offs.

Boy, 4 years, moderately deaf
They just gave me a book, and that was that.

Girl, 5 years, profoundly deaf
They give you a brief chat, but what he did tell me wasn't a deal of use. He just explained how to switch it on and off and how to put the batteries in, and to keep changing the batteries, but beyond that he said nothing. I mean, to stop her getting bits in it, I put it on her back – well they told me at the school that that was useless, but I didn't know. I thought if I put it on her back she wouldn't get her dinner in it – I didn't know that.

Boy, 5 years, moderately deaf
Well they told me how to put it in, but he put it in and when we came out Andrew took it out so when we got home I had to fathom it out myself.

Girl, 1 year, moderately deaf
Well the man that I got it off, he said to make sure they don't chew the wires, and things like that, and to reverse the batteries so they don't wear out one at a time, and they last longer.

Only half of the parents had in fact been given adequate advice on the use of a hearing aid (Table 5.3).

Advice given	Number of children[a]
Adequate	52% (59)
Minimal	29% (33)
None	18% (21)

Table 5.3 Advice given to parents on the use of hearing aids
[a] Applies to the 114 children who had been issued with aids.

Clearly supply alone is not enough if the other conditions concerning efficient and continuous use of the aid are to be made.

(b) *The aid should be suitable.* It is necessary to explain that not all hearing aids are exactly the same. The general public are probably more aware of the concealed type of hearing aids that are more usually worn by the deaf adult. These aids either fit closely behind the ear, or on spectacle frames. However, they are not as powerful as the body worn type of aid, where an ear mould is fitted in the ear and a hearing aid worn on the chest. The aid supplied to children under 7 is the body worn one, because they usually need the extra power, and because the behind-the-ear type is less easy for a small child to wear. There are various types of body worn aids, as aids can act differently to amplify to various extents, and amplify a different range of sounds. The National Health Service supplies two different types of aids, Medresco aids, which are intended to cover the majority of needs.[5] However, where it is deemed necessary, authorities are at liberty to purchase commercially-made hearing aids. In general these are more necessary for children with the more severe type of hearing loss. The supply of the various types of hearing aids is shown in Table 5.4.

Hearing aid supplied	Number of children
Medresco	70% (85)
Commercial	24% (29)
No aid	7% (8)

Table 5.4 Types of hearing aid supplied

The mothers were also asked whether the aid with which they had been supplied had proved helpful to their children. Their replies are shown in Table 5.5 (overleaf).

As will be seen from Table 5.5, a commercial aid was far more likely to be found useful than a Medresco aid. It is unlikely that

Type of aid	Usefulness	Number of children
Medresco	helpful	58% (49/85)
	not helpful	42% (36/85)
Commercial	helpful	86% (25/29)
	not helpful	14% (4/29)

Table 5.5   Usefulness of the various types of hearing aid

this is due to commercial aids simply being superior. It may be that if special trouble is taken to get a commercial aid, special trouble is taken in explaining its use to the parents. It may be that some parents are involved in getting this stronger aid and are more invested in its use when it comes. Alternatively they may be more aware that it costs more, and is harder to get.

Boy, 4 years, severely deaf
This is another thing really, now. It's under, it's a Phillips one, we have to get permission from the Education Committee, and we get the impression that, you know, should we be asking for this type of thing? But we were told at Nuffield, if a child needs it, you know, he's got to have it – a child has priority, you know. 'Cause after all, you think, they're little, they could throw them away, they could do anything with them. We realise we're fortunate, I know. They felt it was needed because Tom hadn't got much hearing, and he definitely has been better with this one, but we do get the leads and that all right. We just had that feeling, we sort of had to get permission first, this type of thing. It's sort of got to come out the rates, you know. It makes you feel as if you're asking for too much, if you know what I mean.

In some cases, though, a commercial aid would be appropriate and the child was supplied with a Medresco aid.

Boy, 3 years, severely deaf
He was promised a more powerful aid. They said they were going to get him a more powerful hearing aid. And every time I went, well they hadn't come yet . . . and they were having trouble with the contract, the hospital was having trouble with the contract or something and they couldn't get them . . . they were very hard to get, so he never did get one.

As will be shown in the last section of this chapter, authorities do differ on their inclination to supply commercial hearing aids, while the degree of deafness within their deaf children does not show the same variation.

For children who found their hearing aid helpful, it could be indispensable.

Boy, 4 years, moderately deaf
He's hopeless without his aid. When I undress him you might just as well not talk to him, and about a fortnight – no, the week before he went to school, it was broke. And I had to take it . . . as it happened we were seeing Miss—— (the peripatetic teacher) on the Monday night, and as I found out it were broke on the Monday morning I took it to her and she kept it and she brought it back about five o'clock on the Tuesday, and he was without it every bit of the day. He spends a lot of time watching telly but he wouldn't even look at telly that day, he was just lost. And then when she brought it back – she brought it about quarter past to half past five time I put it him straight on and his little face light right up. I mean it shows it makes a difference for him.

Girl, 4 years, severely deaf
When we got in I tried it on her, she was tired. No – she didn't want it in, put it on her the next day and I've never had a bit of trouble with her since. She wore it all the next day and every day after that. She only takes it off when she goes to bed at night. If it comes out she comes to me to put it in properly if she can't get it in herself.

Girl, 6 years, moderately deaf
It's not so much that she hears better when she's wearing her hearing aid, but it's easier to get her attention. She seems to listen more readily when she's wearing her hearing aid. Certainly when you speak to her, if she doesn't answer you can suspect there's something wrong with her hearing aid.

For some children, though, the aid did not appear to be any help.

Boy, 4 years, moderately deaf
He won't wear it. He won't wear it now. If he comes from school with it on, it's off – it's slung on the floor, he's never got it on. And if I put it on him – I used to put it on him first thing in the morning, half an hour, he hadn't got it switched on – turn it off or take it off. He's never took to it.

(c) *They should wear the aids continuously.* It is clearly important whether or not the hearing aid is perceived as helpful by the mother.

If she does not think it helps her child, she is less likely to encourage him to wear it. In fact this was often the very reason she gave as to why she did not try and persuade her child to wear his aid.

Boy, 3 years, severely deaf
Well I think if it was of any use he would wear it better, if he could hear with it. If he's got it on he'll wear it, but usually he takes it off whenever he's got the chance, swings the cord about, and he doesn't bother with it.

Girl, 4 years, severely deaf
I can't think she can hear much with it quite honestly. She can hear something because she knows whether it's on or off. She wears it at school but she doesn't show any inclination to wear it at the weekend and if she was getting anything from it she would want to wear it, she is intelligent. She probably hears noise but I don't think it means anything.

Girl, 4 years, severely deaf
I don't bully her about it, because I think if it's any good to her in what she's doing she knows herself whether she wants to wear it or not.

The amount the aid was worn is shown in Table 5.6.

Amount worn	Number of children[a]
All day	52% (59)
Some time each day	30% (34)
Less	13% (15)
Never	5% (6)

Table 5.6   The amount of time deaf children wear their hearing aids
[a] Applies to the 114 children with aids.

The most common reason given for the child not wearing the aid was that it did not seem any use to him, or that he actively disliked it. (Table 5.7).

Attitude	
Dislikes	21% (24)
Varies	24% (27)
Tolerates	55% (63)

Table 5.7   Deaf children's attitude to wearing their hearing aids

Getting the child to wear the aid in the first place had been a problem for many parents. A number of quotes are given here as they may be helpful to parents facing this problem.

Boy, 3 years, severely deaf
—— (my husband) had a fortnight off work, we weren't going on holiday – again it must have been about the August time we had the aid. And—— set out, I can see him now, sitting on the grass. And he kept putting it back, I wouldn't have had the patience I don't think. But he was very good. Until in the end Gary couldn't be bothered any more and he kept it in. And now he wouldn't be without it.

Girl, 6 years, severely deaf
We'd dress up – it was part of the dressing up thing going out with her hearing aid.

Boy, 4 years, severely deaf
It did take a fair while. I just put it on certain times of the day, if he took it off, fair enough. Gradually it just got longer and longer until he wore it all day. Now he puts it on when he dresses in the morning and takes it off when he undresses at night.

Girl, 6 years, moderately deaf
We had terrible trouble at first. I used to get a lot of things out to play with on the table – I used to get everything ready, and whip the hearing aid on quickly and then start doing something – quickly, you know, to get her interest going.

Boy, 5 years, severely deaf
Oh dear, it was very hard work to get him to wear it. Well actually my neighbour did more than we did I think. She played with him and took him for a walk with the dog letting him hold the dog with one hand, and her holding his other hand so he couldn't get to it. Most ingenious really. You know she was a big help. Between us sort of thing, but she was an extremely big help.

Girl, 5 years, profoundly deaf
She wouldn't wear it at first. We used to have to sellotape it in, when she first had it, because she used to keep pulling it out, she wouldn't have it in.

Boy, 4 years, moderately deaf
We'd get him to play with it. We used to play Z-cars.

Girl, 4 years, moderately deaf
It was a bit of a trial at first, but I think I mastered it within a month, which was pretty good going for that age. I used to promise her a lollipop in the summer, or sweets if she'd put it in to go down the road with me to fetch it. So it was in her ear, down to the shop, back and out. That's how I started it. And I'd say – 'Keep it in a bit longer and I'll buy you some sweets soon.' It was lollipops and sweets like nobody's business at first. But it worked. After about a month she was wearing it full-time and not bothering.

Boy, 3 years, severely deaf
I made the mistake at first, you see I didn't know. I've never had anything to do with hearing aids, of just putting the perspex bit in his ear. I thought if he gets used to that, he'll get used to the other part. But on talking to the other mothers I've found that this isn't the best way to go about it. It's best to couple it all up and if it's only for two minutes each time you try, you gain far more than just leaving that piece in, like I managed to one time for forty minutes.

Various reasons were given why a child only wore the aid for part of the day. Some mothers felt that if he had worn it all day at school that was enough, and that it was tiring for him to wear it longer.

Boy, 5 years, moderately deaf
This is where I find it very hard, because you see he's had his aid in all day long and he'll come home from school and usually the first thing he'll do is to take his aid off. He's had enough you see. And you see Mr —— (the teacher) says try and make him keep it in, but he doesn't want to you know. And I think personally if a child goes out to school from nine to four or whatever the case may be, I think that's quite sufficient.

Boy, 3 years, severely deaf
He takes it off at six o'clock, because personally I think he's had enough.

One mother admitted to her husband feeling embarrassment about his daughter wearing a hearing aid.

Girl, 4 years, severely deaf
It worried my husband terribly. Oh he was, he was really – you know. In fact sometimes now, if we're going out somewhere he'll take her hearing aid off.

This feeling may well be more widespread. A child with a hearing aid is conspicuous in this society, and people's attitude to deafness is not always that of sympathy (see Chapter 9).

Other parents allowed their children to decide how much they would wear the aid. They felt to insist on the child wearing the aid was likely to have the opposite effect.

Boy, 4 years, moderately deaf
Well there are people that would have insisted at a far earlier age John had worn his hearing aid. And knowing John this was definitely not on. And now he will go to school at twenty to nine, and come home at four o'clock with it in – you know. Had we insisted at three that he'd worn his hearing aid, would he have worn it now? He's certainly not completely antagonistic to it now. He'll not reject it out of hand.

Boy, 3 years, moderately deaf
I've never insisted on him wearing it, if he takes it off . . . even if he takes it off now I don't try and put it back for perhaps an hour or so. If he takes it off I leave it off. I don't make an issue out of it, at all. Because I think if you insist on it, he's going to go off it more than ever.

Another reason given for not allowing a child to wear an aid all the time was because of the danger of it getting damaged.

Boy, 3 years, partially hearing
I don't let him wear it for rough play because he's gone through so many.

Boy, 6 years, partially hearing
He takes it off when he is playing rough games because he's frightened of breaking it.

This brings us to point (e)

(e) *The aid should be kept in good working order.* With small children who like to play in dirt and water, who spill food, who fall over, who get into fights – how easy is it to keep a transistorised aid in working order? Thirty per cent of parents of children with hearing aids said that this was in fact a problem.

Girl, 4 years, moderately deaf
They're a bit of a nuisance. Either the wire breaks, or the aid goes funny. And the ear mould isn't very good at the moment,

because she was struggling when we took her to have it done. It never has been a perfect fit and her ear's that little bit bigger. So it whistles if you don't put it in dead right, and it's not on full power.

Boy, 5 years, severely deaf
He spills things down it which is terrible because that blocks it. He falls on it – he's so boisterous he's always knocking it. Then he licks and chews and bites the leads in half.

The problem here is if it goes away for repair the child can be without it for some time. On page 105 above a mother described how lost her child was without his aid, and such a story could be repeated many times.

Boy, 4 years, profoundly deaf
The only problem is when it goes in for repair it's such a long while before we get it back. It's been in three or four weeks this time. I think the person who deals with it is on holiday.

Boy, 3 years, moderately deaf
I think their servicing is very poor, in this area anyway. My husband repairs it most times if it's something he can do, because otherwise it has to go up to the Nuffield Unit to be repaired. This might be three weeks, it might be a month. It's very rarely less than that . . . This one he's had it six months, and it's broken down twice but we've repaired it ourselves. They do break down a lot.

This second mother illustrates the option many parents took – that if they were skilled enough they repaired the aid themselves.
One parent was lucky enough to have an extra aid. She had an older deaf child in the family.

Boy, 2 years, severely deaf
The situation is that I happen to have two aids because I happen to have acquired one along the line somewhere. Therefore I can send one away and we've still got the other one. But a normal child will have one aid, and one aid only, and you send it away, and it's ridiculous really – you can lose a week or something.

Certainly with repairs taking weeks and in some cases months, it seems ridiculous that a child should be without an aid for such a time. Even if it was financially impossible to issue all children with spares, one wonders if a central supply of spares could be kept and issued for the period while an aid was away.

OTHER EQUIPMENT

Another type of aid is available – a Russaid. This is a radio transmitter, the speaker wears a transmitter and the child a receiver. This works very well for some children, although they are more bulky than a body worn aid and probably too heavy for continuous use by very young children. No child in this sample was regularly using one at home, though a few were using them at school.

Some mothers had the use of an auditory training unit, or speech trainer. Forty-nine per cent (60) had one permanently, 15 per cent (19) had the use of one occasionally.[6]

Thirty-five per cent had not ever had a speech trainer although in some cases it had been promised.

Boy, 3 years, severely deaf
Well before he went to school, I was promised one of those speech trainers by the Senior Medical Officer. He came to see me and he said he was going to bring one of these machines on his next visit. Well I didn't hear anything more from him for about six months, and when he came again he didn't bring no machine.

Other equipment that four (3 per cent) mothers had, always on their own initiative, was a loop system fitted to their radio or television. This worked in conjunction with the hearing aid and here the child could receive amplified sound through his aid of the radio or television. The cost was borne by the parents.

Girl, 6 years, severely deaf
I've just been writing down here a few notes about hearing aids. It shattered me. We bought a thing called a Magicoil, which is a very small loop system, a local loop system. You put it into the radio or television and then the child puts the other end of this Magicoil into its hearing aid. Sits and listens to the radio you see, and it gets pure reception. The loop system on a coil. Two pounds ten we gave for it and there's less than ten shillings worth of materials – of wire – plastic covering, little plastic box, no it's nothing, and the man that came to fit it on was so disgusted. He said it's just robbing deaf children, he said it isn't as though it's a luxury or an extra for them, he said it's a sheer necessity.

NOTES

1 This, in fact, only applies to minor visual defects, and not major problems of partial sightedness or blindness. The point at issue is the relative expectations of spectacles and hearing aids.

2 For a more detailed discussion, the reader is referred to J. E. John (1964), 'Hearing Aids' in A. Ewing and E. C. Ewing (eds), *Teaching Deaf Children to Talk* (Manchester University Press).

3 HMSO (1968), *The Education of Deaf Children: The Possible Place of Finger Spelling and Signing* (London).

4 In fact it means there is feedback from the earpiece to the microphone. This can be remedied by turning the aid down, or refitting the ear mould.

5 This was the case at the time of the research. The position has now been changed. For up-to-date information the reader is advised to contact the Royal National Institute for the Deaf.

6 This includes five children who had had one permanently but it had been taken away when they started school.

Chapter 6

Learning to Communicate: Education

Apart from equipment, special help for young deaf children is available in the form of teaching. Relative to other handicaps the young deaf child is reasonably well provided for by a peripatetic service of qualified teachers who usually visit mothers and children in their homes though in city areas the mothers and children may visit a central clinic. Ideally these visits are once a week.

Of the parents in this sample, 65 per cent (79) saw a peripatetic teacher weekly. In cases where the child was attending school, their experience prior to starting school is included. A further 20 per cent (24) were visited by a peripatetic teacher less regularly. Occasionally this was once a fortnight, more often it was at irregular intervals. A further 5 per cent (6) had had one or two sessions with a peripatetic teacher. These sessions were purely for the purpose of assessment. Fifteen per cent (19) of the sample had had no help at all in this way.

Sessions with a peripatetic teacher could take various forms. Some parents found the emphasis was on the teacher teaching the child.

Boy, 3 years, moderately deaf
He used to bring games and puzzles, and do things to get him to look. That was the main object, to get him to look at your face.

Boy, 5 years, moderately deaf
It was sensible. I mean it was just showing you games. Probably you couldn't see much point in a lot of it, you know. Hiding things under cups and telling him to tell you which one it's under, but I suppose it was all getting general language into him.

More often though the teacher's role was to show the mother what sort of things she could do with her child.

Boy, 5 years, severely deaf
Basically he came to encourage me. He said he was making progress, even if I couldn't see it.

Boy, 3 years, moderately deaf
She told me anything that I wanted to talk about, she was there to help with the parents' problems in teaching the child, and not so much in instructing the child.

Boy, 3 years, moderately deaf
I learnt off the teacher what to do with Shaun. Otherwise I don't think I should have known how to go on with a deaf child.

Boy, 3 years, partially hearing
He tries to give me guidance, you know. He'll try and give me little things to do with Billy just to see how we get on with them – that sort of thing.

Mothers, while appreciating the teacher coming in and teaching, found it far more worthwhile for the teacher to discuss with them the things that parents could do. In fact most advice to peripatetic teachers stresses the need for them to work with and through the mothers, rather than just with the child. As a report on the work of the peripatetic service puts it: [1]

It has to be made clear that these sessions are for the purpose of helping the parents of young children to understand the nature of their child's disability, and its effects which include lack of normal means of communication. The teacher's role lies in convincing the parents that since facility in spoken English follows progressive stages and can be developed, they have an active part to play. Through purposeful guidance over a period, parents can be encouraged to accept increasing responsibility for this growth of oral language and to make fewer demands on the teacher's time.

One mother went to great pains to point out how much more sensible it is to work through the mother, as she is in a far better position to spend time teaching the child than the teacher.

Girl, 6 years, severely deaf
He was very good but not in the obvious sort of way. I didn't think he was that good to start with, because he didn't seem

to be getting down to anything, but very obviously in the end this was more what was needed. Half an hour or an hour he came for, and in an hour how little he could have taught Janet was really negligible and I think he'd sorted this out. By comparison, the amount he could teach me to teach her during the week was immense.

There are many things the teacher has to get across to the parents. The basic aim of most teachers at this stage is to introduce the child to the idea of communication through the spoken word. Understanding of the spoken word for the deaf is usually through a combination of reading the lip movements and listening to the amplified sound they receive through their hearing aids. One of the important aims then is to get the child to look at the face of the speaker. Here, the teacher who gave advice as to how this could be done, other than just that this should be done, was an immense help.

Girl, 2 years, profoundly deaf
Mrs —— (the peripatetic teacher) – she would give me more assistance as to how to cope with the situation. Whether it's to do with her being a woman I don't know. Like she would tell me, that when I was putting her shoes on to put the shoe to my face and say 'Shall we put Julie's shoe on?' and all this business.

Girl, 4 years, severely deaf
I have to get her to look at my face.
(Q: How do you do this?)
Well I just put her in front of me and try to tell her. I tell her as I would Nicholas, her brother, but clearly, and show her as well as telling her. While I'm telling her I'm showing her at the same time.

One important thing arises from this emphasis on the deaf child looking at the face, for while he is looking at a speaker's face he cannot be looking at what he himself is doing. This means that one very common aspect of mother–child communication is missing, that where the mother describes to the child, or talks with him about what he is doing. It means that any commentary on a game involves interrupting the game. It means that naming objects or pictures cannot be accomplished while the child is looking at them; instead he must hold the image while his mother tells him what they are. Getting used to this can be very difficult.

Girl, 4 years, severely deaf
We've had to teach her to watch. You have to say 'Look', and point to your mouth. There's one thing I did not realise, I used to say 'Look at the cat' and point at the same time, so that she turned round and looked and missed what I was saying, but in time somebody pointed this out.

It also means that whereas mothers of deaf children are often aware that they need to spend a lot of time talking to, and playing with their children, this can be more difficult than with normal children. The interaction required is not a simple or natural one but one which leads to constant interruptions and this makes it more difficult to sustain interest in such games.

As has emerged from the preceding paragraphs, it is necessary for a mother of a deaf child to spend a great deal of time talking to her child. No one can totally compensate for the deaf child missing the incidental conversation which accompanies ordinary everyday activities and is the background to most normal children's lives. However, the more the deaf child is talked to, the more he will learn about language.

For some mothers this came easily. Usually these mothers had talked to all their children and happily gave a running commentary on anything that was going on.

Boy, 4 years, moderately deaf.
I just talk to him. I mean it's no good being silent all the time. You can't. Even if he can't hear. You've got to talk to him really.

Girl, 3 years, moderately deaf
Well I don't stop talking at any time. If anything I talk more. When I'm walking along holding her hand I talk all the time, generally making conversation that you wouldn't do, a running commentary as we're walking. I think I do it automatically. Someone told me the more I talked the better she'll be, so I just talk all the time.

Some mothers acquired the habit out of necessity.

Boy, 3 years, moderately deaf
If you've got a deaf child you probably talk to them more than you would a normal child anyway. Because I don't think the average parent actually talks to their children very much, but if you've got a deaf child you've got to talk to them to make them understand, otherwise they don't hear. So all day long

you're really talking to them, repeating what they're doing and what they're saying, without even thinking about it, so that it becomes a habit.

Girl, 2 years, severely deaf
I didn't talk at first but Mr —— (the peripatetic teacher) says I'm improving now. We go for walks and we talk all the time. If we see anything in particular we stop and look at it, and she looks to see what it is.

For many mothers, to talk to their child constantly was difficult.

Boy, 2 years, profoundly deaf
Earlier I did tend not to speak because I thought 'Well he can't hear so it's not worth it.' But I discovered, of course, that you should talk to them all the time, so now I try to talk to him a lot. It is difficult. Mr —— (the peripatetic teacher) says every time he looks at you you should try and have something to say – in fact all the books say that, but it is difficult. It might be better when Anna's (his sister) at school, because it will be so quiet I'll find myself talking to him I think, like you do a baby. But I did tend before not to speak, it was almost subconscious.

Girl, 2 years, profoundly deaf
I don't find myself talking every day. I've just not got that patience, and it just doesn't come. I suppose if you did keep doing it, it should come natural to you. I haven't found myself making that effort to do it. I do do it sometimes, naturally, but it should be more of a natural thing I suppose.

Some mothers find the whole idea a bit impractical.

Boy, 3 years, partially hearing
The only thing I do find difficulty with – they say you must talk to the child every minute of the day, and they don't take into account what you're doing. Well I don't find it easy to do. If I could go at Neil's pace it would be better, but with other members of the household to look after, and cooking and housework to do, it's impossible. I mean I can't be washing dishes up in the sink and talking to him at the same time. It's probably all right in theory but it doesn't work out in practice.

It must be remembered that talking to a deaf child requires more effort.

Girl, 6 years, severely deaf
It's just more difficult talking to her. You do get used to it, but

even then it is a bigger strain having her sitting up in the evening
than Sharon (her sister). You have to keep talking to her all the
time. It's an effort when you're tired to be patient and to talk.

– and takes longer.

Boy, 3 years, severely deaf
I think this is something to do with the deafness – it takes quite
a while to get things through on occasions. But if I point, which
makes it easier for Paul, he does it quicker, but if I try to make
him spend the time understanding what I'm saying it takes
longer.

As one mother explained – learning to talk to one's child in this
way is a skill.

Girl, 6 years, moderately deaf
I think I realise now – I mean – people say to me, and all the
books you read, and all the people you talk to, carry on about
this business of talking to the child, talk, talk, talk, talk, talk,
to the child. This is what they say. Now this I didn't find easy
and neither did my husband. He probably found it easier than I
did though as I say he misses the exchange of conversation he
would have had with Carol if she'd been a normal hearing child,
but I am not a chattery sort of person. I like to be quiet. When
Carol was occupied with something my attitude was that she's
happy, let's leave her alone. I don't agree with interrupting
children when they're playing. Some people do. I mean, some
people never seem to let them play by themselves, but of course
I realise now that I should have talked to Carol more. This is
a skill, it's a skill I think you've got to learn.

Furthermore, deaf children do not demand language in the same
way that hearing children do, and it can be less rewarding talking
to them. Schlesinger and Meadow describe it thus:

In considering the socialisation process of the deaf child, it is
important to emphasise that he is less likely to provide his hearing parents with the gratifications of parenthood they expect.
The deaf child cannot respond readily to the interaction initiated
by the parent, nor, perhaps, does the deaf child receive the
gratification he needs from his attempts to communicate. While
parental efforts to communicate are not responded to, the less
frequent intrusion of the child's communicative efforts on his
parents have an effect as well.[2]

In the interview situation we tried to discover how much mothers did talk to their deaf children. Of course it would be almost impossible to get an accurate idea of the amount that a mother talked to her child. Rather we tried to ascertain the situations in which she talked to her child and whether she told stories, said nursery rhymes, etc. Sixty per cent (72) of the mothers said that they read stories, or said nursery rhymes with their child. The rest would not go as far as this, either finding it impossible to maintain the child's attention, or feeling that the child understood so little that it was pointless. A further 33 per cent (40) did talk fairly constantly to their children, not taking into account whether the child was listening to them or not, while the remaining 8 per cent (10) only talked if their child was attending to them. None of the mothers said that she did not talk to her child at all.

Also at the interview we discussed the extent to which deaf children liked books and television. Television, and more especially books, can provide a way into the hearing world for the deaf.

The mothers were asked if the children liked watching television. Just over half 52 per cent (64) watched television often; almost every day. A further 32 per cent (39) watched occasionally. Only 11 per cent (14) did not watch at all, and for the other 4 per cent (5) children the question was inappropriate, because of the age of the child, the additional handicaps, or the lack of television.

The mothers were also asked whether their child liked looking at books, and how often they would both sit down and look at a book together. For four children this question was seen as inappropriate because of a combination of their age and/or handicap. Of the remaining 118, 90 per cent (106) liked to look at books and 10 per cent (12) did not. Children who disliked looking at books were evenly distributed throughout the age groups. Two (2/27) in the 2–3½-year-old group, five (5/42) in the 3½–5-year-old group, four (4/34) in the over-5 group. Half of the children looked at books with the mothers at least once a day (39 per cent (46) once a day, 13 per cent (16) more than once a day). Twenty-three per cent (28) looked two or three times a week and 22 per cent (26) did not look often, if at all. Surprisingly, whether a child liked looking at books did not seem to affect how often they looked at books with their mothers. Of the twelve children who disliked looking at books, one still looked every day, five two or three times a week, and six less than that.

Beyond just talk, talk talk, the mothers were also encouraged to put in some systematic teaching of their children, usually to sit down with their child and a speech trainer, a machine which, though cumbersome, provides greater amplification than a hearing aid. Some mothers enjoyed teaching their children.

Boy, 3 years, moderately deaf
He used to have set lessons, he used to love all these lessons but he's past that. He seems to realise now he has enough words to keep him going. He used to have his speech trainer and drag it out, and we'd sit and have a lesson, and I'd be worn out after an hour and he'd say 'No', and he'd say 'Some more' and he'd go on and on and on. But now, I don't know, he just seems to know he's got enough words. If he wants to know a word I tell him what it is, and I write it on his blackboard, and he knows most of these words written down.

Many mothers, however, found it difficult to assume the role of teaching – to sit down with their child and go through some specifield activities with them. To some extent it seemed that the role of mother and the role of teacher conflicted.

Boy, 5 years, moderately deaf
I had a speech trainer brought to the house, and we tried this, ooh for months and months on end, and he just pull them off and throws them. He doesn't want to know, and this is what I tried to put over to the teacher of the deaf. Because I think personally, he (the teacher of the deaf) thinks I'm not trying to help him (Timmy) enough, but he wants to be here and try to do what I do with Timmy, or what his father does with Timmy. He just doesn't want to know. When he gets home all Timmy wants to do is to help his Daddy, or go out and play, or to play indoors.
(Q: Why do you think this is?)
I think, like he'll tell you – Mrs —— (the school teacher) he'll say. Mrs —— is everything to Timmy. You get the book out and say to Timmy 'What do you think?' or 'What does so and so mean, or say?' and he'll say 'No – Mummy no, me school you' he'll say. He knows that he does it at school and that you shouldn't be telling him that sort of thing. Or he thinks in his mind that you shouldn't be doing that. Mrs —— should be doing it. This is the thing with Timmy, you can't get over to him that you're trying to help him as well. He can't see it, and you can't make him understand. If you could just make him understand that it's for his own benefit that his father and I try to make him sit there, but he just won't sit there. If you knew the fights I've had, trying to help him – it's very very hard.

Boy, 3 years, moderately deaf
I think it's hard for a mother to teach. Teachers tend to push this forward – that I should spend an hour each day with him on my own, I mean we have an hour with him each evening with him, as a family, when we get him to say things. They persist that a mother should have at least an hour on their own teaching them, but Michael wouldn't let me do this. I mean I could sit with him for two hours and get little or nothing out of him. He doesn't want me to teach him.

Girl, 4 years, profoundly deaf
Yes. Well they know what they're doing. It's difficult. A child, they'll take notice of a teacher whereas it won't take notice of its mother. It knows it can get away with certain things with its mother that it can't with its teacher and it'll take more notice. You see I couldn't learn her to read and write like they have done there. I could help her a bit, but after so long she takes no notice, she just packs up, whereas at school she can't.

Boy, 6 years, severely deaf
Oh yes, this often happens – oh yes (not liking her teaching him because she's his mother). That's because he's had so much of it from me, from when he was about one year old you see. I started to try and work with him, and things that he won't do for me now, he'll see me in hell before he'll do them, but he'll do them quite happily for anybody else.
(Q: What sort of things are those?)
Well, if I want him to do some maths or something like that or some writing for me he'll work like mad – his reading is on a par with other children of his age and his maths, but he won't do it for me.

One mother made explicit the difference she saw between the role of a teacher and that of a mother.

Boy, 5 years, moderately deaf
I think you should help a child, I'm not saying I don't help Timmy, but in a way that's not schooling. I think the teacher's there for that purpose, and I think you're there to learn them, as I say, to do shoe laces, to do his tie, things in general that a mother should learn her child. I think, anyway, teachers have got a different method of teaching a child.

Another mother explained it differently.

Boy, 2 years, profoundly deaf
I find this very difficult. I always feel that if he weren't my
Francis, it would be that much easier to do it in a formal way.
That's not to say I don't teach him, because I feel the whole
day is given over to teaching him in many ways. But to sit down
with a speech trainer and actually pick up a cow or a bus – this
is difficult.

This last quote, from a mother who was herself an infants'
teacher, points to where the main problem may lie. She herself
distinguishes between two types of teaching, teaching in the formal
sense, and teaching in the sense of providing situations in which
the child may learn. Whereas parents told to teach their child, particularly as this must be sitting down in order to use a speech
trainer, envisage that a formal situation is necessary; conversations
with teachers of the deaf clearly indicate that they have in mind
something far more casual. They see the mother as in a position
to be an ideal teacher in that she can exploit situations as they arise
to allow the child to get as much as possible from them. Of course,
many teachers go to great lengths to explain how they see the
mother's role, and how she can help her child, but from the interviews it seemed that many mothers were left with a feeling of
inadequacy because they were not teaching as they understood it,
and beyond this, bewilderment, because intuitively they felt they
could not combine the role of mother and teacher.
In fact problems did arise when the mothers felt they should
use their play sessions with the child to talk to the child.

Girl, 6 years, severely deaf
Oh well, she's a lovely nature. Very sweet. I like playing with
her, although it is a strain sometimes. It used to be when she
was at home all day, before she started school. I think that with
deaf children, when you play with them, it's concentrated play,
particularly if you're playing in pairs. It's sometimes difficult
when you're playing with them not to concentrate on teaching
them things – you know. Always trying to pack in as much as
you possibly can. You have to be careful not to try and cram
too much in, and let them enjoy playing whatever it is.

Boy, 6 years, severely deaf
Colin and I always seem to be together once Colin's here, purely
because I have always been working with him, do you know
what I mean? And I think if I am perfectly honest with you, I
don't think I could say enjoying it comes into it any more, be-

cause you seem to be conscious all the time as I am pumping enough into him with what we are doing now. I don't know how to put it into words really, because I honestly don't – I mean I am happy with him – don't get me wrong, but as regards saying do I enjoy that, I enjoy taking him to the swimming baths, I enjoy that, but it's a real strain.

It seemed that, for some mothers, if the play situation was used as a teaching situation, this took the play, i.e. the fun out of it. Other mothers, while spending a lot of time talking to, and playing with, their deaf child, felt guilty that they were spoiling them.

Boy, 3 years, severely deaf
He enjoys it. He loves me talking to him. The house used to be important to me, but it isn't now. I would find I was in the middle of doing the bedrooms when it was time to do the dinner because Gary had wanted, you know, he would be responsive and I used to pack in and sit with him. And I've enjoyed talking to him but I've probably done too much of this you see. It made us very close and we had difficulties when he first started school. He didn't want to stay. But what do you do – if anybody could tell me. He's got the speech and now I'm wrong for doing everything else. I've probably tried too hard, but if I started again I'd do the same thing.

Some mothers invented their own technique for trying to get their child to talk.

Boy, 4 years, moderately deaf
He got on my nerves – eh, eh, he used to go. And I thought – well you can talk, because you have talked when you were a baby. I mean he said 'Mum-Mum' and 'Dad-Dad', so I thought – well he's got it in him, he makes all the different sounds, so he can't be stone deaf. Well he usually has about three Shredded Wheat for his breakfast, and of course I only let him have one. And he turned round and he went 'Eh' and I said 'What do you want? Do you want MORE?' and I sat there for half an hour until he said it. He said it in the end and he's never forgot that word.

One may ask why there is all this emphasis on getting the deaf child to talk. In a society where most of those with a significant degree of hearing loss communicate by sign language, one may wonder why parents of deaf children are not taught these signs, so that they may teach their children to communicate. The whole emphasis, however, of all the advice that the parents were given was on the development of the spoken word. The aim is ultimately to facilitate the child's integration into the hearing speaking community. Many professionals in the field of deafness feel that if a deaf child learns to sign, it will inhibit his development in oral language.

> The use of conventional signs, as distinct from natural gestures, gives a superficial impression of good communication and is resorted to by many people including parents, but while it facilitates understanding at a very simple level and at that level could be called communication, it is not really so.
> . . . The use of signs is a very primitive form of language and creates a barrier against correct and fluent communication between adult and the profoundly deaf child; it is an easy way out for the adult and expects very little in return from the child.[3]

> If you want your child to talk in a normal way, you must speak to him as you would to any young child, not in an unnatural manner. If you persist in using gesture or pantomime he will not trouble to learn to talk. He will imitate you and learn that it is easy to get what he wants by gesturing. After that you are going to find it difficult to establish good speech as the means of communication. In order to compete and conform as an adult, good speech is essential.[4]

> It is impossible to recognise the acquisition of a sign language as a good alternative (to spoken language). It is not a verbal language.[5]

> A child who signs 'Bed-me-there' instead of saying 'My bed is in there' is leaving out two important words 'is' and 'in', is confusing 'me' with 'my' and puts bed first instead of second. This jumbled way of thinking becomes so ingrained that if he persists with signs, he will have great difficulty in both reading and writing. He must learn as soon as possible to say complete phrases and sentences.[6]

This view has been criticised by many who feel either that there is no evidence that signing inhibits the development of the spoken language, or that spoken language is so difficult to acquire for the deaf child that he has the right to an alternative means of communication.[7]

Some would argue that learning to communicate by signing can facilitate the development of speech. However, the advice given to

all the parents interviewed was not to develop systematic signs
with their children, and in many cases to exclude gesture as far
as possible. Some parents understood and were in complete accord-
ance with this aim.

Boy, 4 years, moderately deaf
Well, I don't think they should use the signs, I mean if they
can learn them to talk, because if they can get away with signs
they'll never talk. I don't think they use a lot of signs at school,
not to what they used to years ago.

Girl, 6 years, moderately deaf
We've tried to avoid using gesture actually because we want her
to develop her speech. I do tend to wag my finger, which she
copies. We don't use any gestures without speech at all. She is
capable of speech and I think, therefore, we should encourage
her.

Boy, 6 years, severely deaf
It's important for him to use language because we want him to
be able to speak and communicate with normally hearing people.

Girl, 6 years, severely deaf
I think I use gestures more than I should. I think I shouldn't
because they're not sentences primarily – I don't use gestures
without words as well, but if I'm using a gesture it's sort of,
do you want a drink of milk? (with sign). I think this puts her
in the position of not watching my lips enough.

Some parents found it difficult to avoid using gestures with
their deaf children.

Girl, 4 years, severely deaf
They don't like you to sign anything, but occasionally you find
it necessary, you know. When you do it you're only really showing her what you mean. I'm not really gesticulating all the time.

Boy, 2 years, severely deaf
Well using gestures helps us. It helps us to communicate with
them a little bit more with the gestures. But he's not got to the
sort of deaf and dumb language sort of thing, it's just gestures to
show you what he wants and what he doesn't. They tell us at
school 'Try not to' – but sometimes you can't help but do it.
And I mean I've noticed at times that they have to use them.

Boy, 3 years, severely deaf
Well I don't think you can avoid it, quite honestly. I know you

shouldn't and I don't want Gary to gesture. But quite honestly I can't imagine a deaf person could communicate without some gestures. I mean, how do you show them?

Boy, 3 years, moderately deaf
We're told not to use signs at all, but in fact he uses signs, without even being taught them, so we've carried on with whatever he does.

Boy, 5 years, moderately deaf
I try not to, but you sometimes just forget. Especially if I'm doing something, if I was baking or washing and I wanted him to fetch say his slippers or his trousers. Say his trousers to be washed. I'd say upstairs and trousers and do this business (mimes). I try not to, but if I'm washing I forget and I do it.

Sometimes, in particular situations, gesture could seem the only way of communicating.

Girl, 3 years, severely deaf
Yes we gesture because I can't tell when she's thirsty and that. I mean if she wants a drink she's got to tell me somehow.

Boy, 4 years, severely deaf
I don't encourage them because it discourages speech, but some they have to have, you know, like if he wants to go to the toilet.

There did seem to be a general feeling that some gesture at least was necessary. As was stated in Chapter 1, only 29 per cent (34) of the mothers did not use gesture at all to communicate. For some mothers, if their child did not understand the spoken word, they felt they must achieve communication somehow, and gesture was the answer. Mothers do want to communicate with their children, not just because it is useful, but because it enhances their relationship, it brings them closer.

Girl, 5 years, profoundly deaf
You can't just sort of talk. If she does hear any kind of word, it's not a word anyway, it's only babble. I think you've got to communicate that way. I don't care how much they say that you shouldn't. You can't just stand there and do nothing.

Girl, 4 years, profoundly deaf
Oh I don't mind gesture, I think if they can understand anything it's better than not understanding at all. Anything's better than nothing.

Girl, 4 years, severely deaf
I would use anything to communicate with her.

Boy, 3 years, partially hearing
We try not to gesture but I do sometimes. It's difficult you know.
I think you find yourself in situations where you have to. I think
you feel the value of him understanding at that point is probably
better than him learning the words probably.

Of course there are occasions when it is essential to communicate,
whatever the mode.

Boy, 4 years, moderately deaf
Well it's a good thing for one thing. If anyone taps him he can
come and say more or less who hit him. He makes you understand which one it were like. There can be twelve kids on front
and one of them thumps him and he'll tell you which one
thumped him.

Boy, 5 years, profoundly deaf
Well there's nothing else really that we can do, is there?

Boy, 4 years, profoundly deaf
Well we can't really stop him because it's the only means of
communication with him – see if we stopped that and relied on
his voice we wouldn't get nowhere with him. We've got to use
signs to him, though we do try and make him so he doesn't use
the signs.

It can sometimes be necessary to communicate in order not to be
left out.

Girl, 5 years, severely deaf
At one time I was very much against any sort of signing. I
thought it didn't help the speech. But after thinking about it,
because you can't take a blind bit of notice of what they say –
they – because everybody thinks differently, I think, they need
gestures so that they can communicate quickly, otherwise they
get left behind and they don't know what you're on about. If
you can bring – you should be able to bring speech into it, so
that – sort of talk while you're doing it.

Siblings and other children often adopted gestures as an obvious
means of communicating with a deaf child.

Girl, 6 years, severely deaf
John (the hearing brother) has to be reminded of it much more

than I do (using language). I mean I'm better than John, John's aspect, reaction to it is more realistic than mine. I mean it's all very well to go on about language, but basically I mean he's concerned about playing and talking to his sister – he wants to get on with it, he wants to play the game, so if he can give Paula a bash on the arm and say 'That's wrong' he does.

Girl, 4 years, profoundly deaf
She's got to 'gesture' really, hasn't she? It's a case of having to if you want to be understood.
(Q: Do you worry it might cut her off from other people?)
No, because all the kids round here do it with her.

Boy, 5 years, moderately deaf
He talks more when they're not here (the other children). The girls do speak up a bit too much for him. If I say 'Timmy' you know – instead of letting him turn around himself Carol will go up to him 'Timmy – Mummy'. And I'll say 'No, you musn't do that,' I'll say, 'because I shall never know how deaf he is if you keep on doing it.' And they think they're helping, and I keep on at them, and they think – Oh God, she's nagging again. But if they could just leave me alone, I know I could do a lot more with him.

When asked whether they approved of the use of gesture with deaf children 62 per cent (76) of all mothers approved, including three who did not use gesture with their own deaf child and only 18 per cent (20) were categorically against the use of gesture (Table 6.1).

Given that most teachers advised the parents not to use gesture,

Mothers using gesture	
Approve	60% (73)
Disapprove	7% (8)
Not sure	6% (7)
Total	72% (88)
Mothers not using gesture	
Approve	2% (3)
Disapprove	11% (14)
Not sure	14% (17)
Total	28% (34)

Table 6.1   Mothers' attitude to the use of gesture, and actual use of gesture

a finding that 72 per cent do use gesture with their children is surprising. It is also disturbing that many of these parents use gesture despite the feeling they are doing wrong, and the consequent soul-searching and feelings of guilt.

Given that this has been a controversial issue in deafness for as long as there has been an educational policy towards the deaf, one feels that maybe parents need more information in order that they can decide for themselves. There would be problems in this though. One can hardly expect our peripatetic teachers to present both sides of the issues. Being people committed to teaching, we must allow them to be committed to a way of teaching. Furthermore, many parents want clear-cut guidelines as to how to cope with their deaf children. Coming to terms with the consequences of deafness is enough to ask, without having to decide between various points of view on the best way to teach deaf children.

Most parents, in fact, found the peripatetic teachers supportive and helpful.

Girl, 5 years, severely deaf
Its very helpful. You can talk about the progress of your child and things that you probably don't think of or know of that can help you do something else with your child.

Boy, 3 years, moderately deaf
Oh, very good – I don't think Shaun could have been like he is if it hadn't been for the teacher he had – he was that good.

Problems could arise though. Sometimes the peripatetic teacher was seen as doing inappropriate things.

Boy, 6 years, partially hearing
I stopped him coming – he didn't take to that very well. I'll tell you. Well, he was supposed to be teaching Nicholas, well he brings a tea set if you please, well this annoyed me. Well, this is not teaching, I mean Nicholas's deaf, he's not mental, you know what I mean, and it did annoy me that.

The use of a tea set would be regarded as appropriate by most teachers of the deaf. However, it can only fail as a technique if its significance is not understood by the mother, if it is seen as casting aspersions on her child's intelligence.

Some mothers felt the teacher did not take to their particular child.

Boy, 3 years, severely deaf
She used one of these speech trainers with him, and she sort of

E

played with little horses with him, but she did the same every week. She never tried anything different, she just did the same every week. And she had a little roundabout with wooden things on that went round and round. But she seemed to lose interest, you know, because he didn't . . . I think the other children she had, they could speak a few words, he just used to fling the toys and make a lot of noises. She tried to get him to talk into the mike and he wouldn't even do that.

Sometimes, mothers felt the advice they were offered was unrealistic, or did not take full account of their own particular situation.

Girl, 2 years, moderately deaf
They say to sit for a few hours with her, and say words, and keep on saying them and look in a book – where she won't sit for that long anyway.

Girl, 4 years, profoundly deaf
Sometimes it's been sensible and sometimes it's been damn near stupid. I mean Miss —— (the teacher) suggested that to get Veronica interested in the names of things, when you're pegging out the washing, each thing you peg on the line, tell her what it is. Well I could see myself on a freezy cold day out their telling Veronica what each thing was. And I thought stupid! you know.

This second quote illustrates another aspect to this problem. Here it is not the advice which is inappropriate; in fact, it represents sensible advice as an example of the sort of thing the mother might try to do, even if the example given was not a good one, particularly in this case. The difficulty here is that the mother fails to see the advice in the general terms intended, and also feels that the teacher does not appreciate her particular situation. Instead of being a help and support to the mother, the teacher is seen as lacking in understanding and therefore not helpful.

Often a lack of communication between the mother and teacher led to a feeling on the mother's part that the teacher did not fully appreciate her problems.

Girl, 3 years, moderately deaf
I used to have a peripatetic teacher, and I used to say – she can do this, and she can do the other, and he didn't believe me, and that's all there is to it. So I thought I'll prove she can do it, when there's nobody at home I taped her, and she was very clear on it. She does better with nobody listening to her.

Girl, 1 year, profoundly deaf
I don't like going there any more. I don't like the things she says.
One day she says – the last time I went to see her she said
'Oooh she's backward', you know, and I must force her to do
things. Well I don't believe in forcing a child. And I must put
on the speech trainer three times a day, or more – well, once a
day is sufficient, at her age anyway. I didn't take her advice at
all and I don't go.

Whereas some mothers did seem to have genuine grievances, in
some cases it seemed to simply be that you cannot 'please all of
the people all of the time'. One teacher was found over-optimistic
and unrealistic.

Boy, 3 years, severely deaf
I think teachers of the deaf should stop the waving-the-flag
optimism. I think it's unrealistic. And whatever anybody says,
deaf children aren't hearing children.

– while another was off-putting and depressing.

Girl, 5 years, severely deaf
Probably I wanted too much and he's not the sort to give you
any hope, not really. I mean at first, the first words he said to
me when he came round to see me about Heather were 'Your
daughter will have to go away when she's six.' And the first
reaction was, 'No' of course, and then you kind of pull yourself
together.

Often parents felt that the teacher did not understand the particular problems they had with their own child.

Boy, 5 years, moderately deaf
He tried to tell me what to do with Timmy. But I think no one
can tell you what to do, because you do what you want to do
with your own child anyway. But they don't know how difficult
it is. They say they do, but they can't know how difficult it is,
or they wouldn't tell you what to do with them. I do try to, sort
of, as I say help him, but he won't co-operate with you. You
can't get through to him that you're helping him. If you could
explain to Timmy, 'Well, I'm helping you – it's helping you by
doing this such and such a thing' you know, you'd probably be
okay, but he just won't co-operate with you. I can talk to you
because you're research and that, but when I talk to the teacher
I feel guilty. I really feel guilty that I'm not playing my part,
you know. Although I do constantly try.

(Q: Is this because the teacher suggests things for you to try?) Yes, I think this is it. You know they say 'You should try so and so' or 'You could try so and so with Timmy or do so and so with Timmy.' But you can't do that with Timmy, I don't care what anybody says – you cannot do it. That child will not do that thing, you know. The times we've tried, you know, and he's gone to bed and I've cried and cried and cried to my husband. And he says 'Ooh, you're silly.' But I say 'I must try and help him', and he says 'You've done all you can for him, you know.' But I cannot help him, I just cannot help him. I've tried so hard. My husband he says 'You're trying too hard, you're upsetting yourself.' You just can't – I've tried.

It is extremely sad when a mother with a genuine loving concern for her child is made to feel she is no use to him. In fact in those cases where mothers did give up with their children it was often because they were made to feel inadequate – and made to feel it was a job for experts. The following mother is a case in point. Having read everything she could about deafness, and put many ideas into practice, the appearance of a competent teacher on the scene caused her to hand over much of what she was doing to the teacher.

Girl, 2 years, severely deaf
From reading those magazines I've found out how to deal with a deaf child. I asked the teacher about teaching her, but she said it would take me about three years to learn to teach her to lip read.

The job of a teacher of the deaf is complex and difficult. The above quotes point to some of the problems that arise, but overall parents were glowing in their praise of teachers. Of the 103 (84 per cent of the total sample) parents who did receive guidance 66 per cent (68) spoke positively about it. Only 6 per cent (6) were against it. Of the remainder, 20 per cent (21) felt ambivalent, usually they felt helped but at the same time discouraged, or sometimes they just felt neutral – the teacher had done no good but no harm.

Girl, 3 years, profoundly deaf
They've never really given me much advice. They've just done things, and then I've seen if I could do them too. They've never said 'It's better to teach her this way or that way.'

Boy, 3 years, moderately deaf
I don't think we've really had the help that is needed.
(Q: What sort of things would you like to discuss?)

Well it's difficult to judge, because you don't really know what you need to know, but I think that he could do with more intensified attention, I think there should be, for the deaf children, somewhere that concentrates more on their speech.

Seven per cent (8) of the group who received help were positive about the help they had received, but felt they had needed more of it. The need for more help was either because the teacher visited irregularly (only 79 out of 103 were visited weekly) or did not stay long enough.

Boy, 3 years, severely deaf
I got on with her all right, but she only came for half an hour. To start with she would mostly try to get through to him, but on the last few visits we spent most of the time talking.

Boy, 6 years, partially hearing
Mr —— used to come to see me when he turned up, one hour per week if I was lucky, well sometimes he'd leave me standing, and sometimes he would be here twenty minutes then away. He's been coming for a year to see Nicholas.

Boy, 3 years, moderately deaf
I have a teacher who comes supposedly once a week, but it's when he feels like it.
(Q: What did he do when he came?)
Had a cup of tea and went.

Girl, 3 years, severely deaf
She used to please herself whether she came or not.

Girl, 6 years, moderately deaf
She'd sit down and have a cup of tea and talk to me and then go away again – and that was all the assistance I got at that stage.

It is very likely in fact that these teachers were overworked, with a too-heavy workload in a demanding job. However, the impression that some teachers 'only came when they felt like it' hardly helped their professional standing.

The mothers were also asked whether they felt advice was necessary for parents of young deaf children. Eighty-three per cent felt there was a need whereas only 17 per cent felt there was no need. Often advice was seen as essential.

Girl, 6 years, moderately deaf
I don't think it's important, I think it's essential. I think, thinking it over, one of the areas in which it's important to bolster your

self-confidence. Quite apart from the actual physical methods of teaching them words, you do need someone to keep your confidence going – and to keep telling you you're not doing too badly – sort of thing. I think this is a very sore need actually.

Occasionally it was the child rather than the parents that was seen as the focus for help.

Boy, 5 years, severely deaf
I don't think it's the parents, I think it's the child that needs every help. The parents have got each other if they're any parents at all (meaning if they behave as proper parents) if they've got a relationship they've got each other to talk to about all these problems, they should have, to try and iron them out. But it's the child that needs all the attention – in my opinion that is. I mean it's the child that's got the problem and they've got to be helped over it every way they can.

Sometimes there might be a specific reason for needing help.

Girl, 5 years, profoundly deaf
I think it depends on the child partly. If you're having a lot of difficulty with a child I think you need it.

Girl, 3 years, moderately deaf
If she did certain things I wanted to know if it was due to her as a child, or whether it was due to the deafness.

Occasionally parents felt resentful about the idea that they should read advice over how to deal with their own children.

Boy, 3 years, severely deaf
To be quite honest I think we resent it to a certain extent.

In fact the whole concept of giving advice to parents about their own children is a difficult one. Everyone is his own expert on how a child should be brought up. A deaf child presents a strange problem, he is your child but there is a barrier, a barrier of lack of communication. Expert help with an ill child is one thing, concerning a relationship it is much more difficult to give or accept help. The teacher has to guide, to suggest, in an area where the issues are not clear cut. He has to speak with authority but allow the mother to be the expert on her own child. He has to show the mother how to develop better communication with the child, while not interfering or belittling the subtle and complex mother–child relationships. No wonder problems arise. The fact that two-thirds of parents felt positive about their help is an achievement. Most teachers who were condemned by one parent were praised by another. Peripatetic teachers are not wholly good or wholly bad. They have an extremely difficult job to do.

SCHOOL

There is a tendency for young deaf children to go to school before their normal hearing counterparts. In this particular sample 62 per cent (76) were attending school, excluding those attending play-groups. Many parents felt their child did need this extra start.

Boy, 4 years, severely deaf
Well I think it's best for them really, to be quite honest, because they do need – so much has got to go in before anything can go out, and I think the younger the better.

Boy, 3 years, moderately deaf
Well I felt he needed to go. I could have refused but it would have made him worse, because he wants to be with other children, whereas at home he only had one little friend. They could give him more at school than what I could.

Some of the mothers had reservations about whether their children should start school so young.

Girl, 4 years, moderately deaf
Well I think she needs something, but sometimes I wonder whether at this age it's perhaps just as important to have a bit of time at home – now that I've seen how she can be in that holiday with the baby. If the home environment's happy, I think it's as well the child has a good deal of time at home.

This was particularly the case with the mothers of the thirteen children who were away at boarding school. Without exception all these mothers had some reservations about their child going away to school.

Boy, 3 years, severely deaf
Well I don't like it at all. In fact every time he comes home, as soon as it's time for him to go back, I say 'I'm not going to send him back.' I always say it, but I always take him. I know I have to take him, but I always say I'm not going to send him back. They don't seem to be asking any more – oh he has made some progress, a lot of progress behaviour-wise, he has, but he would probably have made the same progress at home, I'm not sure of

that but I like to think he would, but he's not making any progress speech-wise, but understanding is more important than
speech at the moment. But I don't like him . . . The longer he's
there the less I like it, it's so institutionalised. I think that they've
got to learn to live in a hearing world anyway, I mean, if they get
too used to being with deaf people all the time, it will probably
be harder to sort of fit in with the normal world, because it isn't
a normal world there, it just isn't, it's definitely different.

Boy, 5 years, severely deaf
Schools. Well in the beginning I was advised to send Darren to
school because he was at that time impossible, and I realised deep
down inside that it was the right thing, and I didn't want him to
go. And I said 'No – he's too young, he's far too little, and he
should be at home.' And my husband really crushed down on me
then and said that everyone else was suffering, and he was causing everybody's suffering, and therefore he must go to school, and
that upset me, because he has to sign the form, and we had a long,
well many a night rowing and arguing about this and in the end
he won. And he said 'Well I'm going to – he must go.' Well
eventually I came round to his way of thinking, but we still argue
about schools – we have a constant argument.

Boy, 4 years, moderately deaf
Well I didn't like it. I didn't want him to go of course. But he's
got to go, and that's it, and we've just got to get used to the idea.
The only trouble is, you see, there's not enough of them sort of
schools for there to be one any closer you see. Miss —— (the
peripatetic teacher) thought as that was the best one for him, sort
of thing, so I mean. They deal with deaf children all the time
so they've more idea than we have you see.

Various special schools are available. The main division is
between education for deaf children and education for the partially
hearing. These two categories are defined in the Handicapped Pupils
and Special Schools Amending Regulations 1962.[8] The definitions
read as follows:

deaf pupils, that is to say, pupils with impaired hearing who
require education by methods suitable for pupils with little or no
naturally acquired speech or language.

partially hearing pupils, that is to say, pupils with impaired hearing whose development of speech and language, even if retarded,

is following a normal pattern, and who require further education special arrangements or facilities though not necessarily all the educational methods used for deaf pupils.

There are day schools and boarding schools for both deaf and partially hearing pupils. Furthermore, for partially hearing pupils some authorities have special units, with qualified teachers, attached to normal schools, the aim being to facilitate integration with normal hearing children. The type of school a child attends depends on the type of education felt suitable for him, and to some extent the schools available in his area. Children living in rural areas are more likely to have to attend boarding schools, as there will not be enough of them in a particular area to arrange day school provision within reasonable commuting distance. The proportion of the total sample attending the various types of schools is given in Table 6.2.

School attended	
Normal	7% (8)
Deaf day school	29% (35)
Partially hearing day school	1% (1)
Partially hearing unit	15% (19)
Boarding school (deaf)	10% (12)
Boarding school (partially hearing)	1% (1)
Total attending school	62% (76)

Table 6.2   Schools attended by deaf children

It will be noticed that more children attend schools for the deaf than schools for the partially hearing, although overall there are more school places for the partially hearing than there are for the deaf.[9] This is because the more deaf the child, the more likely – in the East Midlands at least – he was to start school before the age of 5 years.

As will also be seen from Table 6.2, 7 per cent of the children were able to attend a normal school. These were all children in the moderately deaf and partially hearing range. For a deaf child to attend a normal school would be esteemed a success by many teachers and parents. However, one cannot assume that this is necessarily so. One parent interviewed felt that her child had been deprived by not being allowed to attend a special school. She felt that the normal school could not give him the specialist attention that he needed.

Boy, 6 years, partially hearing
I want him to be amongst trained teachers because he is getting
no education whatsoever. I want him to go to the Deaf School
at A——.

The majority of children, however, were attending special schools.
Problems arise in all special education, because, as the schools are
specialised, they are few and far between. Whereas the local infants'
school is within the community, both physically and socially, for
the normal child, a child attending a special school usually has to
go outside his area to go to school. The problem of a deaf child
not being part of local friendship groups has been described in
Chapter 2. This, of course, is even more of a problem for deaf
children than for children with other handicaps, because they are
often not in a position to go out and make friends easily.

Another problem that arises when the school is some distance
away is that the mother does not have the same contact with the
school as a mother who goes every day to meet the child, who
knows other mothers of children at the school, and in all probability
her own child's teacher. The mother of a deaf child does not have
this casual contact with the school, and the problem is exacerbated
because her child cannot tell her what he did at school. It is all too
easy for the child to live two unconnected lives, a school life and a
home life. Many parents felt very cut off from what went on at
school.

Girl, 4 years, severely deaf
Once they go to school you don't know what they're doing
because very often you don't take them. When I was in A——
I used to take her and fetch her because we were near the school
and that was good, and I knew what she'd been doing that day
and I could chat to her. That was fine and I liked it. In B—— she
just sailed away in this mini-bus and that was it.

Boy, 4 years, moderately deaf
I don't know whether they're learning him that at school, do
you? We don't know what they do at school, but he's only just in
the nursery class yet. Well they haven't said anything about it –
whether they're just waiting for him to settle down before they
start doing anything about it I just don't know.

Boy, 4 years, moderately deaf
Well I know they're helping him, but they haven't said what
ways they're helping him.

Some schools do use a home-school book, a diary in which the teacher writes about the day's doings for the child to take home, and the mother adds her contribution as to what is happening at home.

Girl, 4 years, severely deaf
Sharon has a book at school and her teacher writes in it what she does at school and then I fill it in at night. And she says it helps her to keep a closer contact with the children.
(Q: Do you find it a good idea?)
Well I do, because I know what she does at school, you see, and, I mean like I couldn't obviously know if she was eating her dinner, and I wrote and asked her and she said that she was and it was all right. Then she had a spell when she didn't and they asked me what she didn't like, you see. Then I can tell her.

Such a book does help to keep the contact between the home and the school, and it has the added advantage of providing meaningful areas of conversation for parent and teacher with the deaf child. If a child arrives home from school full of a painting he has done, this is likely to provide a far richer conversation than a topic artificially inspired by the mother.

In the seven cases where the home-school notebook was functioning efficiently, it worked extremely well. It seemed, though, that many parents and teachers, while liking the idea in theory, did not get around to keeping such a book on a regular basis. There did seem to be an initial stage for the parents when they were not sure what to write, or if what they were writing was not the right thing. Maybe if helped through this, more parents would be able to keep the contact going.

As well as a home-school book, ideally the parents should have regular face-to-face contact with the teachers. They must feel free to visit the school, and welcome when they do go.

Boy, 3 years, severely deaf
Yes, they (the school) encourage you to visit. They say if anything's worrying you, you can ring up. They're very good like that.

Boy, 2 years, severely deaf
I've gone to the school to learn these things. When you go to the school I've sort of said 'Well, what do I do with this, what do I do with that?' and they've said – well they've given me ideas, because, as I say, you feel so inadequate you don't feel you're

doing enough for them. We've found that we were mouthing too much, she told me that. You see I learnt that.

Sixty-nine of the seventy-six mothers who had children at school felt they could visit the school if they wanted to. Not all mothers, of course, avail themselves of the opportunity. Sixty-two had visited their child's school at least once, but only twenty-three had a regular contact with the school. Some parents were precluded from visiting by distance. Many others found the visits they did make were not really worth the effort.

Girl, 4 years, severely deaf
They say come any time but I try and go once a week and collect her, and sort of say 'How's she getting on?' and they say 'Oh well fine' and that's as far as it gets quite honestly.

Interestingly, the group of parents who did not visit included most parents who were themselves teachers. They felt that visiting was, in a sense, interfering or spying.

Boy, 3 years, severely deaf
Mother – but we've never had to (visit the school) have we? You see with my husband being a teacher he doesn't interfere—this is the thing.
Father—I certainly wouldn't want other teachers coming and doing it with me.
Mother – See we don't do it with ——'s (his brother's) teachers.

Girl, 4 years, severely deaf
They say 'Come whenever you like', but you never feel really that you're welcome, you're bound to be interrupting something.

Seven parents felt discouraged by the school from visiting. A number of quotes are included, as the discouragement can be subtle and lie beneath an overt positive attitude to parental visits.

Girl, 4 years, profoundly deaf
(Q: Do you think parents are welcome at the school?)
No. You're told they are. We had a meeting about parents and teachers. Well the headmaster gave us all a little lecture . . . well about some parents don't seem bothered about what happens, and I said 'Well, you know, people just don't like going to the school, interrupting, you know, the classes and all that,' and he said 'Well any time anyone comes to the school they're made most welcome' and that. Any time I've ever been I've felt as if I was intruding.

Girl, 6 years, severely deaf
But I have wished I could have gone into the school on one or
two occasions, I don't mean as a regular thing because obviously
they couldn't do with mothers in and out all the time – you
wouldn't get any teaching done. Seeing how the teacher behaves
with Helen in the class situation with this particular hearing aid
– this I did ask actually if I could, but one felt that this was not
really on. This I think depends entirely on the teacher – I think
the headmaster was quite willing for people to go in, but that
teacher says she's so busy she hasn't time, then he can't tell her
she isn't – and in fact the girl is right, she is so busy – she really
hasn't time. But I wasn't going with the intention of being a
nuisance, it was to sit say for a couple of hours one morning,
keeping in the background, and just watch.

Boy, 5 years, severely deaf
They're very pleased for you to inquire but I don't think they
like you to see the life there. I don't know, I might be wrong but
that's the impression I get. I stayed the first day, I put him to
bed at night, I stayed in the hotel opposite, put him to
bed myself at night. But the headmaster wouldn't let me stay the
next day, and I badly wanted to, just to see the routine and what
they did but he said 'No, ten o'clock's long enough.' So I went
and said good-bye to him at ten o'clock. It was terrible. I'd love
to go. I really would. For a whole week.
(Q: Did he understand when you left him for the first time?)
Oh no. He was four and a half. He couldn't tell. He kept going
to the window and looking at the hotel opposite, he thought I
was there, still.

These problems are there with day schools, but as the last quote
indicates, they are more acute when the child is sent away to
boarding school, and many parents feel a rift developing between
them and their child.

Girl, 4 years, profoundly deaf
Don't see so much of her now. She doesn't seem the same as she
was before she went to school. She's not as interested in me.
Makes me sad in a way.

Although theoretically children at boarding schools are allowed
home every weekend, this was often not possible. Either it was too
expensive for the parents to make the two return trips to the school
to collect and return their child, or the journey was so long that it

could not be fitted in with the needs of the family as a whole. If
the father is the driver in the family, getting the child home may
mean he has to take time off work, and in many jobs this means
losing pay.

Boy, 3 years, severely deaf
I get him home every fortnight. They're allowed to come home
every week, but I just can't afford it. We usually manage . . . so
far I've been on the train only once, we've usually managed . . .
Either my husband's had an afternoon off work, or Mrs A——'s
(a neighbour with a child also at the school) husband has the
afternoon off, and we fetch them in the car. But it seems hardly
worth it. You only get one full day with them at a weekend, you
know. All Friday you spend fetching them and getting back, then
you get Saturday, then Sunday they've got to go back again. So
you only sort of get Saturday and when he first comes home, he's
always a bit withdrawn when he first gets home, as if he doesn't
know what's going on, where he is, at first, and he just gets used
to being at home, being his old self again and he's going back.

Girl, 4 years, severely deaf
Well if we could afford it, she could come home every weekend,
we bear the expense and we can claim from the LCC for fetching
and taking her for holidays and for two weekends a term. Well
the distance it is, to go on the train would cost you over £5.00 to
go there on a Friday and take her back on a Sunday it would cost
over £5.00 and then you can only get two weekends a term
repaid to you, it's an awful lot of money. We'd have her home
every weekend if we possibly could.

Of the thirteen children at boarding school, only five got home
weekly. One child only got home for the school holidays. The rest
got home some weekends, but by no means all. These children
ranged from the ages of 3 to 6 years. They were, with only one
exception, children with very poor language – it is difficult to
believe that they could have had the remotest idea what was going
on. Mothers, in general, were very much against their young deaf
children having to go away to boarding school. Some accepted it
with resignation.

Girl, 3 years, severely deaf
Well it's the only one there is.

When one considers what an upset it would be for a hearing child
to go away from home, how much more so is it for a deaf child,

particularly as at the time he goes away from home he may have been very dependent upon his mother.

Boy, 4 years, moderately deaf
Well I've missed him since he went to school. I've missed him something shocking. With him being deaf you see I spend more time with him, so when he went to school . . .

If this mother missed her child so much, one wonders how much he missed her.

Of course mothers have the right to refuse to allow their child to go away to boarding school, certainly before the age of 5, and beyond that if they are prepared to make a fuss. Not all mothers were aware of this. They also often saw the school as being able to provide more than they could at home, by way of special equipment and qualified teaching. One wonders whether such gains do in fact compensate for all that a child loses when he is sent away from his home. Mothers also have the feeling that if they do not go along with the recommendations made by those in authority, this will be a black mark against them for the future. Some felt that to refuse boarding school would mean to turn down any chance of their child receiving any special education.

Some mothers, usually middle class, were in a position to move home to avoid their child going to boarding school.

Boy, 2 years, profoundly deaf
Round here there's nothing else. In fact we are moving to A——because of this, because there's nowhere for him to go to school, except B—— and that's residential. I don't know why they keep them residential because all the experts agree it's bad for them.

Those children fortunate enough to get to or from school in a day often had long distances to cover. Normally taxi or mini-bus transport was provided as a matter of course, though in one case a mother had had to fight even to get this.

Boy, 3 years, moderately deaf
At first it was either me going by bus every day and fetching him – it's a long way – it would take me as long to get there and back, as soon as I got home I'd have to go backwards and forwards again. It's not as if we've got a car, and apart from that we shouldn't have to. So we asked for a taxi, we've had to push. If it had been for me I'd have thought 'No, we can't have this' but with it being Mark I really stuck out. I'd have gone further than

education, I should have carried on going until I'd have got somebody that would have done it. You've got to stick out. If you don't, I think they do what they want with you.

Given the transport, of the sixty-three children at day school, two were away from home for 9 hours or more in a day, fifty-seven for 7–8 hours, and four less than 7 hours. Although a day of 7–8 hours is normal for a hearing 5-year-old, it must be remembered that many of these children were still only 3 and 4 years old.

Boy, 5 years, moderately deaf
(Q: Does this seem a long day for a child of N's age?)
Not so much now he's six because he would have to go to school for those hours anyway, but when he was three I used to think it was a long time.

Boy, 5 years, moderately deaf
(Q: Does this seem a long day for a child of N's age?)
Well it's not so bad now, but when he first went he used to be the first one to pick up and the last one to drop off. Well sometimes it was gone five before he got here – I used to feel that was too much. (Child picked up at eight o'clock). But now they pick him up last.
(Q: How old was he then?)
About four.
(Q: Did you say anything about it?)
No, the bus driver changed. But really I don't like to say anything about it, because they've got so many to pick up, they have to plan the route the best they can. But I did feel it was too long. He was really tired when he did get home.

Despite all these problems, the vast majority (71 out of 76) of parents did feel the school was helping their child.

A NOTE ON DIFFERING PROVISION

In all the aspects mentioned in this chapter there were variations in provision depending upon where the family lived. In some cases this was understandable; clearly it is harder to provide day school special education in a rural area than it is in a city. On some matters, however, the reasons for such differences are not so clear. The research covered thirteen different areas, and they differed vastly in their provision.

Let us take the provision of hearing aids as an example. In one authority thirteen out of sixteen children (81 per cent) had commercial hearing aids, but in five of the authorities no child had a commercial hearing aid. In three of the authorities all the children had received hearing aids within one month of being diagnosed deaf, in one authority only one-third were supplied within the month, and in another only half.

In the matter of visits from peripatetic teachers, only one authority provided weekly visits for all the children seen; a further four provided weekly or erratic visits for all the children. However, in one authority only half the children had weekly visits and a quarter had no visits at all.

The question of the importance of early diagnosis will be discussed in the next chapter. However, it is interesting to note in this context that of the five children under 2 years in the sample, three were from one area. Clearly deafness is no selector of area, so the conclusion must be that facilities are much better in some areas than others.

In all the aspects in this chapter, authorities differed. This was not, however, systematic. There is no 'best buy' as regards area for the parents of a deaf child.

NOTES

1 HMSO (1969), *Peripatetic Teachers of the Deaf*, Education Survey 6 (Department of Education and Science, London).
2 H. S. Schlesinger and K. P. Meadow (1972), *Sound and Sign: Childhood Deafness and Mental Health* (University of California Press, Berkeley).
3 C. Fry (1964), 'Language problems in profoundly deaf children' in C. Renfrew and K. Murphy (eds), *The Child Who Does Not Talk* (Spastics International Medical Publications).
4 A. H. Ling (1968), 'Advice for parents of young deaf children: how to begin' *Volta Review* No 70, pp 316–19.
5 A. and E. C. Ewing (1964), *Teaching Deaf Children To Talk* (Manchester University Press).
6 D. M. C. Dale (1967), *Deaf Children at Home and School* (University of London Press).
7 J. Denmark (1973), 'The education of deaf children', *Hearing*, Vol. 28 No. 9.
   K. P. Meadow (1966), 'Early manual communication in relation to the child's intellectual, social and communicative functioning', *American Annals of the Deaf*, No. 113.
   S. P. Quigley (1969), *The Influence of Finger Spelling on the Development of Language, Communication and Educational Achievements of Deaf Children* (Institute for Research into Exceptional Children, University of Illinois).
   E. R. Stuckless and J. W. Birch (1966), 'The influence of early manual communication on the linguistic development of deaf children', *American Annals of the Deaf*, No. 111.

8 HMSO (1962), *Handicapped Pupils and Special Schools Amending Regulations*, Statutory Instrument No. 2073.
9 HMSO (1968), *The Education of Deaf Children* (Department of Education and Science, London).

Chapter 7

Coming to Terms with Deafness

In the last two chapters the value of the correct hearing aid and help from trained teachers was stressed as necessary to allow the deaf child to develop to his full potential. All in the field of deafness are agreed that for this help to be most effective it should start as early as possible in the child's life. This in turn implies that the early diagnosis of deafness is important. The official policy of the Department of Education and Science is that children should be screened early in life for possible hearing loss.

It is important that adequate screening for hearing loss of young children, both in early childhood and again when they start school should be undertaken. Ideally, all young children should have their hearing tested.[1]

The view of the Secretary of State for Social Services is that such screening is being carried out.

Health Visitors are instructed in methods of screening young children for hearing impairment as part of their normal training, and it is routine for them to undertake this function. Information is not available on the extent to which children fail to be screened but I would expect the number to be small. Reorganisation of the Health Service will not affect the present screening arrangements except I am sure it will facilitate the general development of Health Services for children.[2]

Though such early diagnosis is the expressed aim of many local authorities, the experience of many parents interviewed in this study did not bear this out. In fact, the major point of concern of virtually all the parents was not the lack of assistance they were receiving at the time of the interview, but the lack of any help or guidance when they first came to think that their child was deaf. Of course for any parents the realisation that one of their own children is handicapped in some way is a time of great sadness. For many parents of deaf children this time was made even more difficult by the rigmarole they had to go through in order to get a diagnosis at all.

Most mothers interviewed had thought that their child was deaf long before it was officially confirmed. For some it was a gradual realisation.

Boy, 3 years, partially hearing
I thought there was something round about six months.
(Q: Why did you think that?)
Well several reasons. One, he was too quiet, he made more of the baby noises, you know, and he had difficulty in locating sounds. He couldn't locate the sources of sounds. The other thing was he didn't seem to recognise my voice which I thought was – he should be doing.

Boy, 3 years, moderately deaf
I had a feeling, yes, because he used to sleep an awful lot, no noise woke him up ever, and if you dropped things like a saucepan lid or anything he never jumped. In fact he didn't jump at all until he was about two and a half years.

For others, there was an inkling at the back of their minds which became a definite feeling because of some particular situation.

Boy, 3 years, severely deaf
I knew there was something wrong – let's put it like this. Having had a normal baby I knew Gary was very withdrawn. I know that word to use now. As a baby he just used to lay there. But he cried a lot as well, he had an odd cry, it was more of a squeal. And strangely enough he still woke to the dustman. Why I don't know. Whether it was coincidence I don't know, but you would imagine a deaf child couldn't hear them. I could vacuum in the bedroom and he didn't wake but then again a lot of normal children do this. The first time, I suppose, that it hit me . . . we had a bouncer for Alison (his sister) in the corner of the room, it was invaluable, and he loved to be in this. And it was a dark evening and the light was on in here. I'd given Gary his tea and he was quite happy bouncing away while we were in the kitchen and I walked through the door, and I said 'Oh, have we left you here all alone,' talking as I came towards him. And he was facing the music you see. We'd got the radio on and as he saw me he

jumped, and he was frightened, and this was . . . I just went weak at the knees.
(Q: What did you think? Did you think it was his hearing or something else?)
At that time I knew it was hearing, then. But prior to that I didn't know whether he was retarded, he did give that impression.
(Q: How old was he then?)
Six months. I remember it clearly. I had suspected it from about three months alone. I hadn't even mentioned it to B—— (my husband) because it sounded ludicrous. It just doesn't happen to your child, does it?

For others the feeling that their child was deaf was triggered off by something specific.

Girl, 1 year, degree of hearing loss not known
Well actually I found out myself. I went to a friend's once for dinner and they've got a dog and it's got a really sharp bark, and she just said to me – 'Ooh she's gone that close to Tracey and she's never jumped' and I said 'Yes I know, we've got an electric kettle and it's ever so loud and she takes no notice,' not thinking, and then when I got home I thought 'It is funny' and I brought in an alarm clock and put it right close to her and she never . . . well you know. And then I asked the doctor when I went there.

Boy, 5 years, profoundly deaf
Well it were the lady next door that told me. She dropped the coal bucket on the hearth, when he was a baby this was, about eight months old, and she says he never flinched. And so we took him to the doctor's.

For others there was a vague feeling that there was something wrong with their baby, although they could not quite put their fingers on what it was.

Girl, 3 years, profoundly deaf
She wasn't chattering away like a normal baby. She was slow in everything. She wouldn't sit up or crawl or anything. I thought there was something wrong, but I didn't know it was deafness. I thought there was something wrong with her mentally, something like that.

Boy, 3 years, moderately deaf
I think I always knew. I think from the time he was born I knew that there was something wrong with him. You know, it was just

intuition. I used to say to my husband, 'There's something wrong with him,' and he would say 'Oh you're mad, there's nothing wrong with him,' and I would say 'Well there is, he either can't hear or he can't see.'

Boy, 3 years, severely deaf
When a child isn't quite normal, they've got that vacant look. Well that's how Daniel was. He was about five months then. He never seemed interested in anything. He used to sit in the pram, but there was no . . . he had this vacant look.

For those babies who had been deaf from birth (91), about half of the mothers realised there was something wrong by the time the baby was 12 months old (Table 7.1).

Some mothers went to the doctor's or their health visitor at the baby clinic the moment they thought there was something wrong. Others waited until they were more sure, testing the child themselves before approaching anyone. Unfortunately the experience of many mothers was that they were just not taken seriously.

Boy, 4 years, severely deaf
The Health Visitor that used to come round now and again, I used to put it to her, because she'd dealt with the other two boys, Tom didn't talk like the other two. Each time I said, she said 'Mrs A——, you're worrying over nothing – he's just lazy with his speech.' And this is what the doctor said as well.

Boy, 6 years, severely deaf
I tried to tell them, I knew straight away there was something the matter with him and I thought it was his hearing when I saw him in the Prem Unit, but then we kept working on it and when he was about five months old took me continuously taking him to the doctors from when he was five months until he was nine or ten months, and to get the doctor to get me an appointment with a specialist. The doctor kept saying I was just a silly mother.

Birth	7% (6)
1–5 months	23% (21)
6–12 months	24% (22)
12–23 months	30% (27)
2 years +	6% (5)
Not until told	11% (10)

Table 7.1   Age of child when mother first thought there was something wrong

It takes a lot of courage to admit to oneself that there is something wrong with one's child. To have it then denied by those in authority can be heartbreaking. For others, the suggestion that they were worrying without any real cause provided a straw to cling to until they were again forced to recognise that there was something wrong.

Girl, 4 years, moderately deaf
I think when she was fifteen months I said to them 'She seems slow starting to talk,' and they said 'She was early walking and feeding herself, you very often find this with babies, they're slow in one thing.' And I think I mentioned again, just mentioned it that was all, about eighteen months. I was getting a bit worried – she did seem slow. I really started to think something was wrong about two years.

Despite all the stress that has been laid on early diagnosis of deafness, the feeling of many mothers was that the doctors just did not want to know. In some cases the doctors were apparently unaware of the possibility, let alone the importance of early diagnosis.

Girl, 5 years, moderately deaf
I kept going to the Welfare but they said there was nothing to worry about, that they didn't start worrying until they got to the age of three.

Boy, 3 years, severely deaf
We'd thought so (that he was deaf) for quite a while (five months). The amazing part about it was that they turned round and said 'It's nice to get somebody you know, as young as this. We usually don't find out until later on,' which amazed me.

Other mothers were told not to worry.

Boy, 5 years, severely deaf
(mother of the child whose deafness was the result of meningitis) I brought it up again and again and I was told that that was the least of my worries at that time.

Girl, 4 years, profoundly deaf
(a mother who already had one deaf child) At seven months she had a hearing test, and they told me both her ears were perfect, and I had to fight to get her another hearing test . . . I had the Health Visitor call, she'd be about seven and a half months, to ask me if she'd had all her injections and the hearing test and

that, and I said yes but I wasn't quite satisfied with the hearing test so she arranged . . . well in actual fact she told me not to be silly, that they'd know their job you see, so I still said I wasn't satisfied, that I'd like another one; so of course they weren't quite sure the second time.
(Q : How old was she then?)
I suppose she'd be about eight and a half months.

As the last quote shows, even when a hearing test was given, this was not always conclusive.

Girl, 1 year, profoundly deaf
I thought she was, when she was a few weeks old – or days. You know when the Health Visitor comes, after the midwife's been and you're discharged completely, at about ten days – well I told her, and she didn't want to know. And then you know when you take them to the clinic, well I told them there. Well they rattled a rattle, but she rattled it there where she could see it so she turned round to see it.

In fact testing babies can be a difficult procedure, particularly with an intelligent baby who may have already learnt to use other cues to compensate for his lack of hearing. Ideally the child sits on the mother's lap while somebody engages his attention to the front. Somebody else then makes various sounds of different pitch and loudness at the back. It is then observed whether or not he responds to the various sounds. This assumes that the baby is engaged in looking to the front, and has no other clues as to what is going on behind him, apart from his hearing.
The age at which deafness was confirmed is given in Table 7.2.

0–11 months	34% (31)
12–23 months	37% (34)
24–35 months	20% (18)
36 months or over	9% (8)

Table 7.2 Age at which deafness was confirmed (excluding those children for whom the onset of deafness was not at birth)

Clearly from Table 7.2 we see that the hopes expressed by the professionals in the field of deaf education for early diagnosis are not met. Two-thirds of the children are not diagnosed until after they are a year old. In some cases this is because mothers do not ask for a hearing test until after this age. The authorities that provided routine screening tests for hearing were in a minority at the time of this research. This routine screening was paying dividends in that the average age of confirmation of deafness was far lower in these authorities than it was in others. The mothers were asked how long it was from the time they first approached someone in authority until the time that they were definitely told that their child was deaf. This is given in Table 7.3.

0–2 months	30% (37)
3–4 months	17% (21)
5–6 months	12% (15)
7–12 months	16% (20)
13–24 months	7% (9)
Over 2 years	2% (2)
Other[a]	15% (18)

Table 7.3   Time between approaching doctor and confirmation of deafness

[a] The other category includes 12 per cent (15) cases where the mother did not realise until she was told – usually these were children picked up by a routine screening test. In a further three cases the mother could not remember when the diagnosis was made.

For just under a third of children deafness was confirmed within two months of the mother approaching the doctor. We can reasonably add to this the 12 per cent where the mother did not realise until she was told. Thus for four out of ten children diagnosis was prompt. The disturbing fact that emerges, however, is that for one in four children it took over six months to confirm the hearing loss, and for eleven out of the 122 children (9 per cent) it took over a year. One or two stories are told here at length to give an indication of what some mothers went through.

Boy, 4 years, severely deaf
I took him to my doctor (at seven months) and he didn't believe me to start with, but he said he'd send him down to the Infirmary, and I had to wait then until Simon was almost fifteen months old before I actually took him to the doctor there.
(Q: What was the delay?)
Well it's just they have a very long list of ear, nose and throat patients.

Girl, 3 years, severely deaf
She was about two months old when we first started to notice that something was wrong.

(Q: What were you noticing – what sort of things?)
Well there was no response to sound.
(Q: What did you do?)
Oh – that's a long story. Well I took her to my doctor when she was six months old and he said that it was impossible to be able to tell, at six months. He didn't think, in his opinion, that there was anything wrong with her.
(Q: On what did he base this?)
Well he banged and he, you know, all this business and he said that some babies won't turn to sound at that age, at six months. Bring her back when she's twelve months, and we took her back when she was twelve months didn't we? and, er – they were still not sure. (To husband) Now how old was she when we first got her to see a clinic, an ENT specialist wasn't it? She was two, wasn't she? She was two when we first started to get something done about it.
(Q: You kept going to your GP until she was two?)
That's it. The last time we went to a different doctor, he was a new doctor in our practice, and he said 'Being as it's worrying you so much the best thing for you to do is for her to have a hearing test at the clinic.' That was the clinic in, no, we went to see Mr A——, consultant at the B—— (hospital), first, and Mr A—— put us in contact with the audiological clinic – this is it.
(Q: And you went to the B—— (hospital) when she was two to see Mr A——?) Yes, and he said children were not his line, he would refer her to people that dealt with children with this sort of problem, so then we went to the audiological clinic.

Parents talked very vividly about what they had to go through at this time.

Girl, 5 years, severely deaf
It was a lot of mucking about. It wasn't very satisfactory, until I blew my top, and then I got something done. That took eighteen months. They just didn't care enough really.

Girl, 6 years, severely deaf
So really it was four and a half before deafness was eventually diagnosed, but all the time you see Mum has to push, push, push. Really it all began at ten months, the opportunity was lost then, you see deafness, no matter what you've trained for, deafness is something that if you've never met it, you've never had it in the family which we haven't – if you've never come across it except in the street – that's old people who you speak to slowly who have

had years of speech training – you don't understand it, you don't know what it means.

Of course the assessment of hearing loss is not clear cut. In some cases the child was given some sort of assessment. One mother of a very bright little girl took over two years to get proper diagnosis, because her little girl *seemed* so normal on superficial acquaintance.

Girl, 4 years, moderately deaf
When I went to the Welfare a bit upset saying I was sure something was wrong, that I had to see the doctor there, and they said if it would make me feel any happier they'd come to give her a hearing test. Then I had second thoughts and rang the Social Worker up and said 'Don't bother' – and she said 'It's no bother. If it gives you any peace of mind we'll come.' So they came – did it. I didn't think it was very satisfactory. It just showed up everything I'd worried about. You couldn't get her attention. She seemed to hear – but you couldn't keep her occupied for very long – she'd be wandering off while you were talking. And they said she was too young to test, but they thought she was all right, and they said to come back in six months if I was still worried, so I did that again you see.

– and nearly two years after the first visit

They asked what vocabulary she had at two and a half see, and I listed lots and lots of words and they just went by pure figures, that number of words was quite acceptable for a child of that age. And I said 'Yes, but it's not so much the words, it's she doesn't understand what I try to tell her, she's never with me really.' And they said 'Come again in six months if you're still not happy', which would have been when she was about three, but before she got to three, a few months before, I just couldn't stand it any longer. I knew something was wrong and I had to have a bit of a show down then to say 'You either try and find out for me, or tell me where else to go this time.' I went round intending to really find out something that time and she said 'Come the following week when the doctor would be there and she'd fill you in', because I could explain a bit more at that age as to what her troubles were. And I wasn't in there very long on that occasion. The nurse went to talk to Jane herself, being older – 'Would you like a sweet, Jane?' from this distance with Jane's back to her. I said 'You're wasting your breath.' She said 'Why?' I said 'You've got to tap her to get her on our level, and just say "Sweet" – that's all she understands' and she said 'Don't you think she's deaf?' And I had an appointment for the next week, and four hospital appointments in the next month and things really got moving.

Here is another example of a similar problem.

Boy, 4 years, partially hearing
No, I wasn't told. I told them, actually. Well Peter was a rhesus baby, he had seven exchange transfusions at birth plus one normal one. And of course I had to keep taking him back, every week at first, and then every fortnight, and each time, well not each time, nearly every time, I kept saying he doesn't seem to hear very well; and they never took any notice, and then one of them said 'You've mentioned that a lot of times now, I think we'll better just check it.' Well he got a cup and rattled it – well with Peter being a rhesus baby, when I went to these appointments there was always several people in the room because it's a teaching hospital, and he was looking everywhere, and of course he watched the cup. And they said 'No, of course he's not deaf', and so this went on for several months, and he kept saying 'We must do something about this, because you keep mentioning it again', and I said that he was not turning round when you spoke to him, and he just didn't take any notice of you, unless he could see you, and this bothered me. Then they said 'Right, we'll make an appointment for an audiological clinic' and he had an aid.

Boy, 3 years, moderately deaf
I wasn't told, I told them, and they didn't believe us. We knew at nine months; Ray at nine months, you could shout and shout and he couldn't hear. We took him to the ENT specialist, and he said he could hear. We took him at thirteen months and he said he could hear but he thought perhaps he had a slight loss.
(Q: And he still wasn't responding?)
Nothing at all, I mean we *knew*. There wasn't any point in arguing about it. We lived with it, it was so obvious. It wasn't as if he was a partially hearing child, he just did not hear. (Diagnosis finally made at nineteen months.)

Clearly this sort of problem in diagnosis usually happened in cases of a less severe degree of hearing loss. In general it was not these sorts of problems that upset the parents most. What they did find very hard to bear was just not being taken seriously by doctors and others. When a mother, after a deal of heart-searching, takes the big step of going to a doctor to say that her child has something wrong – to be dismissed as a worrying neurotic mother is just

Satisfied	65% (79)
Dissatisfied	23% (28)
Neutral	7% (9)
Don't know	5% (6)

Table 7.4 Mother's feelings about the way she was told about her child's deafness

tragic. This whole area is beset with problems. On the one side you have professionals emphasising the importance of early diagnosis and early auditory training, and on the other, mothers feeling there is something wrong with their child and help not being forthcoming. For mothers this creates problems. It is hard to admit one's child is deaf, and harder still to maintain this position against the 'experts'.

When the time actually came for the confirmation of the deafness, most mothers felt the doctors did as well as they could under the circumstances (Table 7.4).

The doctors (or teachers) were seen as having a difficult job which many performed with sympathy and kindness.

Boy, 5 years, severely deaf
We took him and saw a specialist. And we were there a full hour and he gave him the works. He was marvellous, he really was, it was a thorough examination. And he explained in detail.

Girl, 6 years, severely deaf
I don't honestly know if people could have done any better than they did. I think the medical men at A——, excluding Dr B——, who has now left, he was good in his way but he was of the miserable medical school, he told you all the terrible things he'd diagnosed and didn't give you any hope for the future. But the other people we've met since have been absolutely marvellous. They did what they could.

Where people complained it was usually about the bluntness of the approach.

Girl, 3 years, profoundly deaf
Yes he just said those three things, he just said 'She's deaf, backwards and got a deformed head. Next.' – you know. It was horrible.

Boy, 3 years, moderately deaf
He asked me first of all if I thought he was deaf and I said, you know, I had a slight thought that he might be. He just turned . . .

we were both there and he just said 'Oh your son's got to wear a hearing aid in one ear, we think he's a deaf.' Rather lax I think in the way they did approach it. They didn't offer any help or advice, anything like that, he just said 'Ricky's deaf.' Full stop . . . and go and see the audiologist in the hope that he can supply one.

It is not an easy matter to tell parents that their child is handicapped and it may well be that a blunt approach is necessary for some doctors and some parents.

Girl, 5 years, severely deaf
I knew really but I wanted somebody to tell me. But not 'Of course you know your daughter's deaf.' I didn't want this. I wanted a roundabout and – say, well you know, er, nicely. Although deep down I knew it I suppose.

Boy, 3 years, moderately deaf
I don't think they can tell you any other way. Really I think you've got to be told blunt. It's no good trying to cushion it. They just told me straight out that Alan was deaf. You can't cushion a thing like that really.

In some cases deafness was never confirmed to the parents.

Boy, 5 years, moderately deaf
Nobody really told us that Timmy was deaf. Not what you'd call really confirmed it. This is what annoys me. I've never really had confirmation that Timmy was deaf. I always feel sometimes you'll talk to Timmy and he'll answer, and another time you'll talk to Timmy and he just ignores it altogether. I'm sure there's something that's just slightly wrong that can be done.

Girl, 4 years, profoundly deaf
Nobody actually tells you that. I mean (an older deaf sister) she's ten, and they've still never said 'Well she's definitely hard of hearing', or 'She's deaf', nobody actually tells you that. They just carry on. They have the hearing tests, another one and then another one and then they say 'Well I think she needs a hearing aid' and 'Would you like to have her fitted with a hearing aid?'

For many the actual diagnosis was a relief, after months of sus-pecting, and hoping against hope.

Boy, 4 years, severely deaf
It was quite a shock, but it was better knowing. It was awful, those few months not knowing. That was the worst part.

Girl, 6 years, severely deaf
I think it was a relief to hear somebody say – yes she is deaf – it took away the question mark about why she wouldn't talk.

Girl, 4 years, moderately deaf[3]
I was just sheer relieved to know that it wasn't me going mad, at first. So many people had stood in my path and said 'You're whittling, you're worrying – there's nothing wrong with her, she'll talk when she's ready,' I thought that if it went on much longer at home and that child was supposed to be normal, I'd go off me rocker. So really it wasn't so much finding fault with anybody, or how it had been handled it was just a relief to think at long last we did know that there was something wrong, and what it was, and could tackle it. I didn't know how to handle her before that, I can't really find fault. I wish really that they'd taken more notice when I'd first asked them when I was first worried, but I can see their point of view. She'd got a certain vocabulary. There must be hundreds of mothers with first babies that worry over everything they don't do when they should, that they've got to really sweep with a broad brush, and say – well, come back.

Other mothers found the diagnosis a relief because they knew something was wrong but not what. For these it was a relief just to know, or in some cases to know that it was not something more serious.

Boy, 4 years, moderately deaf
It came as a . . . well I thought perhaps there was something the matter because he weren't . . . well I'd had two before and I know no kids are the same, but he was completely different. He never used to play with boys, he was more interested in knocking things down, you wouldn't get him to sit down and play with anything, he was ever such a strange child. He wouldn't talk. He wouldn't go to nobody, only me. Not even his Dad. I wouldn't say I was shocked but I was glad it was that and nothing else.

Boy, 3 years, severely deaf
Relieved to tell you the truth. Because I was worried that they would say he was retarded to tell you the truth. This was another hurdle we could have done without, another handicap we could have done without. I would have preferred just one or the other.

Boy, 3 years, severely deaf
Well I think the fact I'd realised this before. I think in a way, rather than – I don't know whether it's awful to say this or not,

but rather the fact that he should be mentally retarded it was a relief in a way that it was deafness, at least I felt we might get somewhere.

The mothers were asked when they thought was the best time to be told that a child was deaf. Almost all (93 per cent) thought the sooner the better – either for the sake of the mother or for the sake of the child's education.

Boy, 3 years, profoundly deaf
As soon as possible. I mean you don't want to go on believing he can hear when he can't, do you?

Boy, 5 years, profoundly deaf
The sooner you know, the better you can cope.

Boy, 3 years, moderately deaf
Well, for the child's sake I think it ought to be found out very early because I mean they do such a lot, and then again you get used to it, don't you, you know what I mean. It's a waste of time. Right from when they're tiny as soon as they can fit a hearing aid they can be hearing things, can't they. I mean Mark really was quite old. But of course I kept thinking it was just my imagination.

Girl, 3 years, moderately deaf
As soon as you find out. Mind you there's a lot of people what have had deaf children and they've not known. And kiddies what have gone to school, and they've not been learning at school, you know. I think, any mother that's got a child, especially like Elizabeth was, you know there's something wrong.

Of course not all mothers felt this way. In particular one or two looked back on the time before they knew that their child was deaf and wished it could have been longer.

Girl, 2 years, profoundly deaf
I don't know really. I suppose it's best to know as soon as possible although I enjoyed the time, looking back, when I was ignorant of the fact, obviously. I often think back, and wish I was back in those days when I didn't know anything about it. Because when they're babies they just act and react normally and you don't jump to the assumption that there's anything wrong – you don't think it's going to happen to you – do you?

In the main, though, parents want to know, and to know the truth. Many parents were full of praise for somebody who had sat down and explained everything to them. No parent praised anyone for 'shielding' or protecting them from the truth.

Boy, 1 year, degree of deafness not known[4]
I would like to know the results, because I'm so anxious, I'm a person like this. I like it if there's anything wrong I like them to tell me, I would rather they tell me because then I can accept it and I can live up to it, and know definitely about it, and then I won't worry . . . If there's anything wrong I like them to tell me the truth, but if they try to hide things from me, now that is what I don't like, because that upset me and I get worried, because with my doctor when I first took him there he never told me anything and I was ever so upset. I don't know, but I was ever so terrified when I come home, and my husband had to quieten me down because he wouldn't tell me the truth you see. He never told me anything at all about his heart or his liver or anything, he only just said that the baby was really ill and I had to get him into the hospital. But when Dr A—— told me what it really was I wasn't so terrified, because I can accept it and I know how to look after him. I try my best to keep him cheerful and happy. If they don't tell me I feel terrified but if they tell me the truth I'm broken-hearted and then I cheer up.

Boy, 4 years, moderately deaf
Well I think . . . When I saw Mr A—— (ENT specialist) he never told me nothing, I asked him and he ehed and ahed. I had to take Karl down to see Mr B—— and he told me exactly what he was doing, why he was doing it and the result of it. Now I think that way you can settle in with it . . . you can take it in a bit more, whereas just being left in the lurch, well you do, you dream up all sorts of things.

Boy, 2 years, severely deaf
I think – I'm young, I've got two other children, but he means that little bit more to me because I've got to fight for him, and I think they should put you on the right basis to start with. Say that he's profoundly deaf. I mean I wasn't told until I went to the school that he was profoundly deaf. I mean I just thought he was hard of hearing. I think to myself that with things like this they should put it to you the quickest way, so that you know what you've got, and what you're up against, so we know the position. So you're not sort of thinking 'Oh well I can't be bothered, something's going to happen later on and they'll clear it all up and he'll be normal.' I mean now I know in my heart I know

F

there's nothing. Maybe in years to come they might be able to do something, but at the moment they can't and I've got to help him all the more. I mean I've thought that and now I'll go to the school once in a while.

Whatever parents may think about how they were told, and when was the best time to be told – when it comes to the crunch it is they themselves who have to cope with the realisation that their own child is deaf. Some parents clearly find this more difficult than others. For some it is a sudden shock; others come to realise the implications of deafness more gradually. Many parents, on their own admission, did not initially realise what deafness would mean – in day-to-day terms.

Boy, 6 years, severely deaf
We knew really, but I was heart-broken, we knew when he was being tested it was a shattering time that was, it was terrible but the thing is you just have to keep telling yourself and make yourself try and accept it. The thing is I don't think you ever really do fully, fully accept it. I'm always waiting you know for one morning I'll get up and Colin will be all right, if I was dead honest about it, but really I know he won't be.

Girl, 2 years, severely deaf
No we still don't believe. We are hoping for her. Until about two months ago she couldn't walk at all, and we thought she wasn't going to walk at all, and we'd have to buy a wheelchair for her, and suddenly she started to walk. Until she was a year old she couldn't sit up for herself and they thought she might never sit – and now she sits. So one day it might happen with her hearing. I think she might, you know, develop her hearing.

Girl, 3 years, severely deaf
Well, if somebody had come and said 'She's stone deaf' I shouldn't have known what to do. I was living, hoping like it was one of those things you have to go through and then find out it's not true. I'm still living with it, trying to think that it's not true. It was a shock really because I didn't really believe it. I thought she was probably being awkward.

Boy, 3 years, moderately deaf
It's upsetting. I mean now. That's why we didn't answer your letter before because we've had two or three from one thing and another. It's all right to go and write it down, but when you're not in that kind of mood it churns inside you, do you

know what I mean? It upsets you. Well I knew really. It upset us a lot, and it took a lot of getting over – the silly things you have to get over about him having to wear a hearing aid, you know what I mean, daft things like that. Now I couldn't care less whether anybody sees it or not, but just that instinct, that they're sort of looking at you, but then it doesn't bother you and you just think 'Oh blow'.

Girl, 2 years, profoundly deaf
No, well I still think I tend to bury my head in the sand a bit, you know, even now, although we've known for a while. You tend to think – perhaps it will all be all right in a little while, but you realise it won't. Because it's not noticeable at this age you see, is it – you can excuse her not talking. But it's when she gets older, and you realise it will become more noticeable. I think it will hit me then more, when it becomes more noticeable.

As this last mother points out, there can be two ways in which the realisation is gradual. Firstly, one just does not realise at first what the implications of deafness are, and secondly, behaviours which are acceptable in a small child, not talking, not taking 'No' for an answer, are certainly not acceptable and seem strange in an older child.[5]

Once a mother has come to terms with the fact that her child is deaf, very often she feels a very strong need for more explanation. What caused it? Is it curable? What about an operation? It seems particularly important that the future prognosis be discussed with the parents and if, as in the vast majority of cases, there is no cure for the deafness they should be made aware of this. Many parents had always at the back of their minds the hope of a cure.

Boy, 4 years, moderately deaf
I want to have it explained a bit more. I mean I know all about the inner ear, and the outer ear, but I want to know why Karl's deaf, whether it's a nerve or what. I mean A—— (a neighbour's child), she's partially deaf, she's got fluid in the ear but she can have that done. Now I'm wondering whether something like that could be the same with Karl.

Boy, 4 years, moderately deaf
I don't think they know quite whether it can be put right. I'm building my hopes, that it can be put right.

Boy, 2 years, severely deaf
We thought there might be something the doctors could do. An

operation, or something like that, but they didn't tell us. I think the thing was with me, I thought to myself 'Oh well it could be tonsillitis or adenoids', I mean you hear of so many. I didn't know how deaf he was. I knew he was deaf, nobody told you. And you hear that many people say 'My son was deaf and he had this or the other' and you think that's what's going to happen to my boy, and he'll be all right. But now I know it won't.

Girl, 3 years, moderately deaf
I would like to know on the medical side, can she have adenoids and tonsils out, will it help her with her speech. Is there an operation? No one ever seemed to look deeper. They just said she was deaf, so we'll teach her, but not look deeper into it to see if there was anything else other than deafness.

As time went on the medical profession, looked on as a focus for special help, was often found to be wanting. In some cases the parents felt they had been poorly advised by their doctors.

Boy, 5 years, moderately deaf
It was confirmed at eighteen months but the doctors led us to believe that they couldn't do anything until he was about three. He did have checks on his ears, but at that time they said he would have to be about three before they could do anything.

Girl, 6 years, severely deaf
Well we felt that doctors hadn't known enough really to tell us that she was deaf. But I do realise that it is very difficult but I think that they ought to have told us a bit more. I think they ought to have said 'Well we think she isn't deaf but keep an eye on it,' rather than 'She is definitely not deaf.' And of course you're so eager to believe them that you think she can't be deaf.

In other cases parents felt that the doctors had just not given enough time and attention to their particular child.

Boy, 5 years, moderately deaf
Quite honestly you're the first person I've been able to talk to. Welfare people like the Health Visitor and that – to me they don't do nothing. They do nothing for me. They come round my house. Really all they come to see is if you're clean, or you're dirty, quite honestly that's the impression they give me. They've given me no help, and I refuse to have them in the door. They don't want to listen. Now you're supposed to be asking me things which you have done, but you're also listening to my side of the story. You try to tell people things and they look at you as if

you're stupid. They're going to help Tim and this sort of thing but they do nothing. You go to the hospital, they stick something in his ear, and they say 'I'll see you again in six months' and you go back six months later and they say the same thing. Now to me this is ridiculous, it really is. All these months that's going by and going by, my son's getting older and older and older. And he's getting no further. He's not getting on the way I want him to get on.

Boy, 3 years, partially hearing
The specialist, we go to see him once a year. That is the biggest farce from here to kingdom come and back again. It takes us about an hour and a half to get to the hospital. After we've waited for about half an hour or an hour, and you walk in, and he'll say 'Oh hallo' and Jeremy just goes into his shell, and he won't say a word, and you can't get anything from him, and the specialist will say 'Are you satisfied with him?' and I'll say 'Yes, thank you.' And he'll say 'I've had a letter from his teacher and she's satisfied with him. Come back and see me in a year' – and that's all there is to it. I'm exaggerating. He looks in his ears, but you know, it lasts about two minutes all told.

Girl, 4 years, severely deaf
We sat and waited for an hour and a half and then whizzed in and whizzed out. He peeped into her ear, and said 'Nothing there.'

Boy, 5 years, moderately deaf
I didn't get very far with the specialist I'm afraid. It annoyed me really, more than anything. Well he'd ping this tuning fork and stick it near his earhole, and he'd say 'See me in six months' and this was it. I was getting nowhere sort of thing.

The most common complaint about doctors, however, was that they were evasive – that they would not tell the parents the nature or outcome of their investigations or take them into their confidence.

Boy, 5 years, moderately deaf
This is it. They never tell you nothing. This is what annoys me with hospitals and doctors, and all these things. I think you've got a right to know. I mean he's my son, and I think I should know everything that goes on with Timmy.

Girl, 4 years, severely deaf
Well, they don't really tell you a lot. They write it on the report. They never really tell you a lot, just if she's better than last time.

Boy, 2 years, severely deaf
We've found that you can sit there and talk to them, and they won't actually tell you anything. We took him for a test for him going to school, and that was the first time they told us that they might not be able to do anything for him. And that was the first time, and we'd asked and asked, but they wouldn't say anything to you. And they give you the idea that, when you start first talking about it with one, they give you the feeling – you're on a high cloud, that there's something that might be done. They give you that impression but they don't say it.

This last mother was in the difficult position of having her child brought through meningitis in hospital and feeling it wrong to be complaining to doctors who had saved her son's life.

Boy, 5 years, severely deaf
In the hospital I was rather amazed that there was this complete indifference. This did upset me a good deal because I don't think they could appreciate . . . well all right, they'd done a great deal for this child they'd brought back from the dead twice, and he was getting better, and as far as they were concerned that was a job extremely well done, full stop. And my bone of contention was: well good heavens, there were plenty of specialists in the hospital, why on earth couldn't they refer him to someone else in the hospital, or at least write on a note to my doctor that I'd at least suspected this and could he follow it up. That's what really upset me. Because at that time I was in a terrible state. and it seemed to be the last straw. It is the hospital that I found to be extremely indifferent.

In fact when she had said to the doctors that she thought the child was deaf, they had said (see p. 151 above) 'That is the least of your worries at the moment.' Of course with a child very seriously ill, this may have been the case, and it may be that after meningitis a child may seem different, but she did feel she had not been taken seriously.

Of course one cannot lay all the blame at the feet of the doctors. They are busy people with many other important responsibilities. A routine check-up for them is just that – there is no time allowed for discussion. Parents say doctors do not tell them things, but do they ask? It may be that the situation is such that the parents do not feel encouraged to ask many questions; it may also be that they do not know how to get across what it is they want to know. The problem here is that parents feel they should not bother the doctor with what may seem minor problems, or that their questions may be stupid, or they just do not know what they want to ask.

Another problem is that people may remember what the doctor said to them in a selective manner, that often they remember afterwards only the things they wanted to hear. If a parent desperately hopes for a cure for their child's deafness, whatever is said to them, this hope may still remain in their minds, with minute snippets of conversation to back it up.

The biggest complaint of mothers is however the perennial one that they are not taken seriously. They do know their own children, they are with them all day, every day. We need very good reasons to discard their experience simply as indicating they are anxious mothers.

When mothers were asked who had taken trouble to explain, 8 per cent (10) mentioned their doctor, and 9 per cent (11) their hospital specialist. As might be expected, most help was received from teachers; 38 per cent (36) felt helped in this way. Three parents mentioned other people, health visitors, etc., but the most disturbing finding is that 43 per cent (52) felt no one had really tried to explain to them adequately what the problems were.

Apart from information and support from professionals, there are other sources of help available. The National Deaf Children's Society has many free booklets, and a free quarterly magazine, and local groups of parents in most areas who meet to hear speakers and discuss their problems with each other. There are books, occasional television and radio programmes, and support gained from just knowing other mothers of deaf children. Sixty-nine per cent of mothers had made a positive attempt to get information from one or more of these sources. The parents' evaluation of the usefulness or otherwise of the different sources is shown in Table 7.5.

The NDCS were in fact reaching 57 per cent of mothers with their magazine, *Talk*, and many found it helpful. There were some criticisms, some found it too optimistic, but overall it was a great source of support.

Boy, 5 years, severely deaf
The *Talk* magazine I find marvellous. I enjoy that, I think that's very good because the one thing that you want is – you want encouragement. Even though obviously all children are different and all children aren't success stories but it's nice to know that some children succeed over the handicap and it gives you a terrific incentive to carry on. I enjoy the success stories, and the problems – behaviour problems. I read a marvellous article in

	Information received	Useful	Not useful
Talk magazine	57% (70)	66	4
Other mothers	53% (65)	51	14
NDCS booklets	43% (52)	47	5
Books	37% (45)	38	7
TV or radio	29% (35)	27	8
NDCS meetings	14% (17)	17	0
Other meetings	6% (7)	6	1
Other[a]	19% (23)	22	1

Table 7.5   Information about deafness received by mothers of deaf children, and its usefulness

[a] This includes mothers who received the John Tracy course, a correspondence course free to mothers of deaf children, available from John Tracy Clinic, 806 West Adams Boulevard, Los Angeles, California 90007.

Talk three years ago, and I only wish I'd read that when Darren was very small. It dealt exactly with his behaviour problems that I was experiencing. It would have helped me to understand.

Knowing other mothers of deaf children was another major source of information – though here mothers were more ambivalent as to its usefulness. Some found it helpful to discuss their common problems:

Boy, 3 years, severely deaf
I think it's helpful just being able to talk out your problems without even having any practical help from it, just being able to talk it over with someone – to know someone else has had the same experience.

Girl, 4 years, severely deaf
Well I think you need to get together like, because I think a lot of people perhaps feel a bit lonely, but I think once you're all together and talking about it you feel a lot better in yourself, rather than keeping it to yourself.

Boy, 4 years, severely deaf
Well, yes, because we discuss things amongst ourselves. I think you need someone with the same problems as you – definitely.

There could be problems in discussing with other mothers though. They felt that children were so different there was not much to be gained by talking about them – and sometimes it could be depressing.

Girl, 6 years, severely deaf
(Q: Do you find this helpful? – referring to knowing other mothers of deaf children)
Not particularly. I would like to say yes and feel that we were all in the same boat but all deaf children are so different and of course, we as people are all different. And their ages are different. They're inclined to regard your child as in competition with theirs, it's still the same old feeling.

Girl, 6 years, severely deaf
It can be worrying at times because they (other parents of deaf children) have often such different ideas, which can seem to be the right ideas the way they put them forward and can end up getting you very worried. I think everyone has very definite views on how to bring up their own deaf child and I think with deaf children they're much more definite about it than . . . put it that way.

Girl, 4 years, moderately deaf
There's one (mother of a deaf child) I've seen now and again at the shops. I knew her daughter went to the same school, and I do bump into her now and again.
(Q: Do you find this helpful?)
Not really, because that mother has got all her pieces to tell you. I think that people aren't interested in what your problems are when they've got a child of their own. They just see their own little problem, and theirs is different to yours, and I don't like to talk about it and dwell on it, because you probably come away hearing something ten times worse.

Booklets and books were the next most useful source of information, although for many parents this is not an easy way to cope with information.

Boy, 4 years, severely deaf
They're (books) sometimes a bit hard. I often skip pages.

Other parents found books depressing, either because of the picture they painted of deaf children, or for the amount it seemed that parents were expected to do.

Girl, 2 years, profoundly deaf
I think I found them more depressing than anything. There again it's only trying to bury your head in the sand a bit, but I did find it more depressing than anything.

Boy, 5 years, moderately deaf
The books upset me. They made them out to be freaky.

Boy, 3 years, partially hearing
I think sometimes they make you feel a bit guilty, because you think – Oh I'm not doing this with my child – should I be doing this?

TV and radio programmes, although probably an easier source of information, had not put out many programmes on deafness at the time of the interviews (1971).[6] Programmes that were mentioned were discussions on 'Woman's Hour', the 'Tomorrow's World' programme that had an item on hearing aids and the appeal for deaf children on the children's television programme 'Magpie'. The potential for television as an educative medium in informing people about the problems of the deaf is stressed in the following quote.

Girl, 1 year, profoundly deaf
Well the only television programme really about deafness was when they had that Magpie appeal – appealing for money. I cried on one programme where they showed you what a deaf child can hear. They turned the sound down to nothing and then they turned it up so you could just get one tone, it went hard in that did. That programme – I'd accepted the fact that she was deaf, but until I actually saw it – it hit hard.

NDCS[7] meetings were found helpful by those parents who had been to one, as were meetings arranged by other organisations. Most parents found once they had taken the initial step, meetings were friendly.

Girl, 6 years, moderately deaf
When we finally did decide to join the Society we were notified that there was a parents' meeting and we went to it fully expecting to go as you do to most of these things. To go, sit there, not know anyone, listen to the talk and then come home, but we hadn't been there ten minutes before someone came up and said – we haven't seen you before, who are you, sort of thing – why have you come? He was the Chairman, Mr A——, and we explained that we'd got a deaf child and that we wanted to join the Society and that sort of thing, and the very next day Mrs B—— (the Welfare Officer) came on the doorstep – and said you know – that I've been told that you're newly discovered parents of a deaf child, what can I do to help? – which we thought was fantastic. I mean – we've never really looked back since. I think it was the very next day.

Of course for many parents distance and/or lack of transport was a limiting factor. It is really, though, the initial step that is the hardest – going to a strange place where you do not know anyone. Some parents seemed to feel reluctant to take this step because it would mean them making a positive statement about their child's deafness; others because they felt the time to be better spent at home.

Boy, 4 years, moderately deaf
I don't know whether this has been a mistake or not but it would be wrong to say we haven't got round to it, but we didn't – we haven't become involved with the NDCS or anything like that, I don't know if it's been a misconception on my part, or if you know – we've preferred to do it on our own. I think no one will know John any better than we will. Fair enough, the problems in deaf children who are born deaf must be fairly common, I'm not denying that, but the kids have then got their own personalities which will develop even with deafness, and I think for that reason we've tended to be a bit insular. I don't know whether it's the wrong thing or the right thing.

Boy, 5 years, moderately deaf
We had the chance to go to a meeting tonight, and you'll probably say I'm a bit ignorant but I didn't want to go. I don't think it will help.
(Q: Can you say why you feel that?)
It's just something I have. I can't explain to you why. It's not that I'm selfish or anything, it's just that I don't think it's going to help me or to help Timmy. Because I live with Timmy I could go to a meeting any day of the week, but that means I've got to leave my children from say half past six to about half past eight, nine o'clock, when I could be sitting here with Timmy and my children, you know. And I could be doing something. To me that's a waste of time.

Many parents did feel that they had not been able to find out all they wanted to about deafness, despite the number of possible information sources.

Boy, 3 years, moderately deaf
I think that it's not neighbours or friends you want help from. It's somebody like a Health Visitor, but who knows about deaf children, who could come round and offer some help. You don't want sympathy, you want concrete advice, even if you don't

accept it. You want concrete suggestions and practical ideas. I think looking ahead they could sort of say 'Oh well, in six months' time expect a certain reaction.' Everything lands on you in the dark. This frustration and tantrums, you know nothing of this until it happens. And I think there should be at least one person in an area who can visit, well with any abnormal child really, not just a deaf child, because you are entirely in the dark.

Girl, 2 years, severely deaf
I'd like more information about the future of deaf children in general. Although it did say a little bit in the book, but – it tended to talk about the crafts they could do, and this sort of thing. Well what I really wanted to know was—if they were intelligent whether this would be wasted or whether it would be used – their potential.

Girl, 2 years, severely deaf
Yes, because it's not that the children are just deaf, it's not that they just can't hear. You need to be told about all the background, what it means really. It's not like blindness where they can't see sort of thing – that's all there is to it, that they can't see, but if you're deaf . . . I mean it hadn't occurred to me so much really until recently. I know blindness, there's a lot, not being able to see I mean, but it's a more straightforward handicap.[8]

Another complaint was that although it was possible to find things out, set things in motion, it was the parents who had to make all the effort.

Boy, 3 years, moderately deaf
It's very long-winded, it all seems so . . . it's a load of red tape to get through, it's as if you're going round and round in a circle, and getting nowhere. Well it's been like that from the start. It's sort of . . . it's been such a long drawn out . . . you know, you go from somebody to somebody to somebody until you get the right one. A lot of the time you go round in circles, and you feel you have to push for things you really want.

As most mothers said, the time when you first find out is when you most need help – otherwise one can feel really left in the dark.

Girl, 5 years, severely deaf
Well it wasn't until about three weeks ago I knew even what partial hearing was. (Child had been diagnosed partially hearing for three years.) I didn't know and it was a bit of a shock to learn what partial hearing is. So really I think any parent could

do with a bit more . . . social really isn't it? I think you could do with it more, when you first find out, you could do with it an awful lot. This is why if I found any mother with a deaf child that's only just learnt I would go and talk to them or they would come round, because I had one lady come round not so long ago, and she'd just found out that her son was deaf. He was two and she'd given up hope. Two! and given up hope. Nobody had cared enough really. And this is what I wish – if I knew somebody that had got a deaf child when I first found out. It would have helped tremendously.

Boy, 3 years, severely deaf
Oh I think you do, especially to start with, when you first find out they should automatically . . . if they haven't got the time to explain things in detail themselves they should automatically put you in touch with people who can, like the National Deaf Children's Society, but they don't even mention it. Even my Health Visitor never told me about them, and I mean she had got the time, because she spends hours talking. She'd come and spend quite a good deal of time with you, and she did have time to tell me, but she never mentioned it.

NOTES

1 *The Health of the School Child* (1964), Report of the Chief Medical Officer of the Department of Education and Science for the years 1962 and 1963 (HMSO, London).
2 Reply to questions put to Secretary of State for Social Services on the screening of pre-school children by Health Visitors by Mr Redmond on 23 January 1973, reported in *National Deaf Children's Society Yearbook and Accounts* (1972–3).
3 This mother's relief can well be imagined when it is realised that she is the mother of Jane (see p. 155 above).
4 This was an immigrant family.
5 See also p. 201 below.
6 Recently there have been more, notably BBC2 'Horizon: The Curtain of Silence', 25 January 1973, and ITV: 'Sunday and Monday in Silence', 29 May 1973.
7 National Deaf Children's Society.
8 Although people who work with the blind would disagree with the idea that blindness is a straightforward handicap, this quote does make the point that deafness is not simply not being able to hear.

Chapter 8

Family Life with a Deaf Child

The literature on the care of handicapped children suggests that because of the handicap fathers may participate less in the care of their child than fathers of normal children. In this research the same questions were asked about father participation as were asked of fathers of normal children, and fathers of cerebral palsied children. An assessment was made of how much the father was involved in the day-to-day care of the child, and how much he played with his child, taking into account the opportunities. The results are given in Table 8.1. Certainly there is no indication that fathers of deaf children are any less participant than fathers of other children:

	Highly participant	Fairly participant	Non-participant
All deaf children	58% (69)	40% (48)	2% (2)
Deaf 3·6–4·11 years	65% (26)	33% (13)	3% (3)[a]
Normal 4-year-olds	51%	40%	9%
Cerebral palsied under 7 years	50%	38%	12%

Table 8.1 Father participation with deaf children

[a] Three children did not have fathers or 'acting' fathers at the time of interview. Two of these were in the deaf 3·6–4·11-year-old group.

Of course there were disagreements between parents as to how things should be done. A chief area of disagreement was that of discipline.

Girl, 3 years, moderately deaf
I'm stricter with the children. He doesn't see much of the children, and he doesn't punish them when he is here, and they know it, and they will try and play one against the other. When she's dropping off to sleep, she calls him and he'll go and play with her, when she should be quiet. If he just waited that minute or two she'd drop off, and after a long day you're so grateful when they do drop off.

Girl, 4 years, moderately deaf
Well I suppose he must disapprove of the way I really lose my temper at her. I think he'd handle her differently if she was left in his control completely, but there again I don't think she'd be so obliging if she were given in to. We don't sort of argue over her. I think he realises that we've got some sort of problems and we both try our best. I can't criticise his way because he's easy going, and he doesn't really openly criticise me. He says sometimes that I ought to calm down a bit.

Boy, 5 years, profoundly deaf
Well he says I smack him far too much. I ought to talk to him. Well when I have spoken to him, he shrugs his shoulder and turns his back on me – just walks off and perhaps does it again. And I keep saying to Pete, well you're not with him all day, like I am. And he doesn't do naughty things when Pete's here. Perhaps, you see he likes cars and if Pete's tinkering about with his car, Derek's there you see – and he'll let Derek undo a screw. Well all these things Derek likes. Well my work's the same routine day in day out and I think perhaps he's bored with it. Well if he's got something interesting to do he's not naughty, he's good.

Girl, 4 years, profoundly deaf
He thinks I don't make her do enough, he'll say 'Oh she's spoilt,' and I don't see that because she's an understanding child. If you tell her to do something and you tell her why, she'll do it. There's never any need to be that firm with her, and to me that's enough, you know. I'd sooner she understood what she's got to do, than do it just because I say so. He tends to take the attitude that they should do it because he says so, that he's the father, and they should do it without question, and I don't agree with that.

Many of the parents put forward the view, not that there was disagreement between them over aspects of bringing up the child, but

that they both brought different approaches to the situation and that
these two approaches were complementary.

Girl, 6 years, moderately deaf
Often I can get her to do things when he can't. I think it's
because he does play with her a great deal, and she knows that
he does, and I think that she expects him to be in this role towards
her all the time. Not to be the disciplinarian. It's a pity in a way
because it makes Mum seem like the big bad ogre, but there it
is – I mean . . . we can't both have the same approach. I think
this is inevitable, it wouldn't be right if we did. She needs variety
doesn't she?

Boy, 2 years, severely deaf
We don't disagree, but we bring different aspects to it, I think.
I tend to be far too soft, and he tends to be the other way, in
my opinion. I think this is a good thing. On the one occasion
you need the one, on the other, you need the other.

An area where fathers did have difficulty, and feel embarrassment,
was in trying to talk to their deaf children.

Boy, 3 years, severely deaf
Well I think he should have more um . . . he should be encouraged to lip read more, and you know . . . He'll play with
him a lot, but he won't sort of, try and show him what a thing
is – tell him the words for objects, you know, the names of
objects; and try and impress upon him, 'this is called a ball,
and this is called that'. He would rather communicate with him
in any other way that he could, but not by trying to learn him
words. He'd rather play with him, like—playing ball or pushing
him on the swing, or hide and seek. He likes to play hide and
seek. I would try and find opportunities to get him to watch
me, to lip read, to try and understand what a thing is. I like to
tell him words more.

Girl, 1 year, profoundly deaf
I've had to tell him that he must talk to her. There are times
when he's just acted dumb, and he's made signs and all that.
I've really had to tell him that he's got to talk to her. He's
embarrassed to do it. And with the speech trainer, he wouldn't
speak to her. So we talked it out, and one day while I was out
he plucked up courage and talked to her. He had to make an
effort. He was embarrassed talking to her like that. He finds it
easier now.

Some mothers also voiced the opinion that through being out all day, fathers just did not understand the problems.

Girl, 5 years, profoundly deaf
I think it tends to be a strain. Particularly when they're small. I don't think a man understands quite the same.

It was felt important to establish whether having a deaf child affected a marriage. Obviously this can be a very sensitive area, and very difficult to probe.[1] In some cases it was not appropriate to put the question because of changes in marital status.[2] In certain other cases the interviewer felt that such questioning could prove disturbing to the parents; where children were present at the interview the question was not asked. In one or two cases it was felt unethical by the interviewer to ask about the marriage – for probing in such a way always presents the danger of bringing to the surface problems that are not apparent to those concerned. For this reason in twenty-two interviews the questions about marriage were not asked.

The question was raised initially in very general terms.

Some people say that having a handicapped child brings a husband and wife closer together, and some that it puts a strain on a marriage.

What do you feel about this?

Even when the question is asked, the form of it allows the mother to opt out; rather than giving a personal answer she can make a general comment about hypothetical effects.

Boy, 3 years, moderately deaf
I think any child can bring a family closer together or can put a strain, because you tend to argue over children more than anything else, and I don't think this would apply more to a handicapped child than the average child.

Girl, 4 years, severely deaf
Well of course it could be a strain having a deaf child – it depends on the marriage.

In four interviews a general question was given and the matter was not probed any further. Although to opt out would seem to be a middle-class privilege, of the four mothers who did this, two were middle class and two were working class. The replies given by the remaining ninety-six mothers to the question of the effect of the deaf child on the marriage are given in Table 8.2.

Closer	23% (22)
Strain	24% (23)
Varies (sometimes closer, sometimes strain)	25% (24)
No difference	28% (27)

Table 8.2   The effect of the deaf child on the parents' relationship

Many mothers spoke vividly of the ways in which the deaf child had strained their marriage.

Boy, 4 years, profoundly deaf
Well I think it is a strain – you know. We do get on each other's nerves a lot more than I think we would do, you see when Matthew's got the down I take it out on him (the husband). We do have a lot more to put up with.

Girl, 6 years, severely deaf
It's imprisoned us. It's made us do a lot of quarrelling, not that we didn't quarrel before but it's increased horribly.

Girl, 3 years, severely deaf
I think we argue more than we need do, don't we, because of the strain. It does put a strain on a marriage, definitely.

Girl, 4 years, moderately deaf
I think whenever times of trouble crop up, that's when you find . . . I think I show the signs of strain, and it shows with my husband as well, and if I'd got a happy-go-lucky child that I'd got no worries over I'd be more relaxed with everyone. But you see I get short-tempered, and then the strain shows with his family – I suppose they can tell that I'm not myself again, so that it affects everybody in some way or another.

Girl, 3 years, moderately deaf
I should say it's a strain on a marriage. I should say it depends on the couple, on the parents. My husband like . . . when he's concentrating he doesn't like it broken, he doesn't like his line of thought broken. He works out things down to detail, he likes solitude, he likes to be quiet, he doesn't like to be interrupted every five minutes when he's in a book – things like that, or when he's working out an account. Well you do get this, and therefore – I don't think he's ever really smacked her hard. He's never smacked them in temper. He loses his temper, he shouts, but he's never hit them in temper, but he often wishes he didn't have the bother of them. He doesn't regret having children.

There's one thing he doesn't like, always having to . . . we've never been quiet, but to be on your guard all the time he doesn't like that, he likes to go out and just enjoy himself in the sense that it's free and easy, and children could come along and enjoy it, but Lisa wants attention all the time, and she doesn't let you relax, there's no relaxing at all, till they've gone to sleep.

One parent described how the situation had affected their sex life for a time.

Girl, 6 years, severely deaf
It does at first (affect one's marriage) it certainly did when my husband was very upset. I think we were nearer to a divorce then than we have ever been. When he found out – now this wasn't at the very beginning from my point of view, it was at the beginning from his point of view. And certainly I even think he felt a sort of revulsion – the idea – well he said so. He even went as far as going to the doctor about it, the thought that he didn't want to risk having any more children. I don't think he was consciously worried about it, but um-m he didn't want to – oh dear – he didn't enjoy the idea of sleeping with me any more. I think basically because of this, tied up with this – at that stage I could easily – I don't think he really wanted much to do with me at that time even, we were certainly further apart at that time. We didn't have much to say to each other. I didn't think I wanted anything in particular, it was a very difficult time. No one could help because they didn't seem to know what I was on about. I think that certainly is a very difficult time.

Although this was the only time this came up in the interviews,[3] conversations with teachers of the deaf indicate that this is a problem for at least a proportion of the parents, and the example cited is probably not just an isolated case.

Many parents felt the child's deafness had acted on their marriage in both ways – that it had been a strain, but also that it had brought them closer.

Girl, 6 years, moderately deaf
I think it brings you closer together. I think, quite honestly, any shared disaster – if you could put it not quite as high as that but anything, any trouble really, provided it isn't between you, tends to bring you closer together. I think it also – there are times when you get irritable, irritated with each other, because you're tired and worried which at times we are. I mean, I'm a terrible

pessimist, and my husband is a confirmed optimist. It usually works out all right in the end, but there are times when you find it hard to see each other's point of view – but we always reconcile our points of view.

Girl, 2 years, moderately deaf
I think it brings us closer together in the way that we work together a lot more to help her, but then it's a strain when she plays up, and he's saying 'Oh, you've got to go along with her,' and I've had it all day so I've had enough of it, you know, it's a strain then.

Boy, 2 years, severely deaf
It's a hell of a strain. It's a strain in every sense of the word. It's a physical strain, it's a strain on your own resources, a strain on your joint relationship. But it's also bound to bring you closer together in the sense you're forced to go into things more deeply and analyse them more closely.

And there were those parents who felt their child's handicap had definitely drawn them closer together.

Girl, 4 years, profoundly deaf
I don't know whether it's Samantha but I think we're more in love now than we ever were. I don't know whether love grows in marriage. You see, you don't really know, because you don't compare anybody else's marriage to your own, do you. I mean we love each other – it's not driven us apart I'll give it that.

In the last chapter it was again emphasised that if a deaf child is to develop language he needs a great deal of individual and concentrated attention. As any mother knows, dividing oneself between various children in a family can be difficult in normal circumstances. What happens, then, with a deaf child who is in need of special attention?

Boy, 5 years, profoundly deaf
They don't like it very much, but it's just one of those things.

Boy, 3 years, moderately deaf
Yes. I've had to be very careful. You know when we've been doing anything with Shaun, we've caught Pamela looking, and we've had to bring her in quickly. She has got jealous, it's no good saying she hasn't. Sometimes she's said 'You love Shaun more than me.' We've had to overcome it, it's not so much of a problem now because we catch it while it's there.

Boy, 3 years, moderately deaf
Yes, you've got to give that bit extra. I don't like to do it in front of them (the other children), but they should understand. They didn't like it at first but they do now.

Boy, 3 years, severely deaf
I try not to make the difference, but Paul automatically gets more attention from me because he needs me more. You see Peter's always been very independent – at eight months old he didn't really need me – he was very grown up for his age.

Girl, 4 years, severely deaf
Yes I think so. Not all the time, but I think sometimes I'm inclined to, I think. Janet knows like, Sharon has to have more attention. We've explained to her, you know, that she has to have a bit more attention because she can't hear and Janet's very good with her.

Sometimes the problem can arise from needing to give the child special attention in order that he can communicate.

Girl, 6 years, severely deaf
If we're in the car, you see, and if Janet talks, if Janet wants to know something, well you talk to Janet, you have to look at Janet, whereas you can talk to Becky without seeming to give as much attention to Becky. And if they're both talking at the same time, Becky will get a bit cross and say she started first and so she ought to finish. And it's difficult for Janet to pick up this sort of cue, you know, perhaps even that Becky is already talking, and that leads us into a bit of difficulty sometimes.

When children are away at boarding school there is the problem of when they come home for weekends.

Girl, 4 years, severely deaf
This is a real problem with us because Nicky's away for a fortnight, home for a weekend, away for a fortnight, home for a weekend. Well, for the fortnight Helen has me every time she wants me because there's no one else wanting me, and then for the weekend Nicky needs me so much because she's been away, and Helen thinks, naturally, that she's the one, that whenever she cries she can come to me, and they won't be nursed together, they won't be loved together, and I try to make up to Nicky for what she misses with being away and I try not to let Helen feel that she's been pushed out, but I'm sure she does feel it, because often when Nicky's home she wakes up more at nights, and we

sit together at night, Helen and I, and she has ten minutes' cuddle, I don't think we can do anything about it, except trying to avoid having them both upset at the same time.

Again, problems can arise because the deaf child is the focus of special attention from people outside the family.

Boy, 3 years, severely deaf
I don't think she really understands. It's only recently she's said to me 'I wish Gary wasn't deaf' and I say 'I do as well Sarah, and we have to help him this way', and this is it. Sarah's very sensitive, she understands, but I don't think she understands fully. We try and include her in everything. We always had. This is another thing, with you being here. It's about Gary.

Boy, 3 years, severely deaf
Well Peter's going through a little bit of a difficult period because I had to leave him for a week (on course with Paul) and he was quite naughty with my sister that was looking after him, and at the moment I'm having to be very tactful and make a lot of fuss of Peter to get him over this. This is something he's gone through before you see. When they notice a child's, say, not normal, the child automatically gets more attention because you've got to spend more time with them. Another instance with Peter, I go to a mothers' luncheon club once a month at A—— and I've told him about this, I've told him what we do. And one day he really got me convinced that he'd got this awful tummy-ache. He even looked pale, and I took it in, and I said 'Oh well, you'll have to come with me Peter, you'll have to see what it's all about.' And he was that fit when we got there I thought 'Right, you little stinker, you've seen it now, and I won't fall for this again', but I think it was just his way of finding out where I was going to and what was happening – what he was missing you see.

There is also the fact that the handicapped child may be treated as special by other members of family or close friends – particularly grandparents.

Boy, 5 years, profoundly deaf
I mean I said that he was deaf, but they (the grandparents) wouldn't have it that he was deaf, they said he was slow on speaking. But you see, they perhaps would only see him on Sundays for a couple of hours where I'd see him all week. Well now they accept it, and in fact they spoil him. They think you

can't do enough for him, he plays on them you see because he knows he can get what he wants from them.

This of course can work the opposite way, that other people can leave the deaf child out.

Boy, 4 years, severely deaf
My husband has two sisters which are both married, and I think sometimes they tend to, shall I say, shut their eyes to it, they don't really want to know. And you see if they talk to Christopher they say 'Hello' and then they turn the other way and carry on doing something else, and if Christopher goes and touches them, which he does when he wants you to pay attention to what he wants, they don't seem as though they have time for the child to express what he wants.

Overall, parents did not feel that other members of the family and close friends treated their child differently from other children because he was deaf. In 64 per cent (seventy-eight) of the cases they thought no difference was made. Twenty-six per cent (thirty-two) thought more fuss was made of the deaf child, 5 per cent (six) less fuss, and 5 per cent (six) that it varied depending on the situation. There is also the discipline situation which tends to bring comparison between the deaf child and his siblings into sharp focus.

Boy, 2 years, profoundly deaf
Well, mostly I tend to say to Elaine – 'Well let Miles have it' because he makes the most frightful noise if he can't have what he wants – if he really wants something. And he won't give in you see, and you can't say to him 'Well let Elaine have it for a bit, and then you have it.' That's what I'm coming up against really now. And if he wants some sweets you see, and I just say 'No', when really what I mean is 'Not now, after tea', you can't say that to him, and he thinks you're saying 'No, you can't have any at all.' He cries then you see. And it's the same with toys. Elaine has to give in rather a lot. It's a shame really I think, but you can't get through to him that it's later. He usually only wants it for the moment and once he's got his own way he doesn't want it any more. I put my foot down sometimes and he just has to cry.

Or some mothers just feel protective towards their deaf children.

Boy, 3 years, severely deaf
I suppose deep down I do, but I wish I didn't. I am inclined,

when they're fighting, to expect Peter to stand anything Paul (the deaf child) hands out but to stop Peter if he's getting a little too rough with Paul. (Peter is younger than Paul.)

The mothers were asked whether they made special allowances for the deaf child. Of the 106 with a deaf child and another child of appropriate age[4], over half (58 per cent/sixty-one) found it necessary to make concessions to the deaf child. A further 3 per cent (3) made concessions to the deaf child in some circumstances, but in other circumstances made concessions to other children in the family – to even out the balance as it were. The other 40 per cent (42) mothers made no concessions in either direction. Far fewer mothers of deaf children felt able to make no concessions than mothers of cerebral palsied children interviewed in a similar study.[5] Here 51 per cent found they did not need to make concessions.

Some mothers found that, because they made allowances for the deaf child, they modified their behaviour to other children in the family accordingly.

Boy, 3 years, severely deaf
You can't do the same with a deaf child. You do bring them up differently, you've got to, but at the same time . . . It also makes it that you bring the other one up differently, because you've had to give in to Gary a little bit more so I'm probably giving in to Sharon where I wouldn't normally.

Of course jealousy is not always manifested directly, but in oblique ways.

Boy, 3 years, moderately deaf
Yes I quite often get the sort of remark 'Well Michael's had it' or 'Michael's got it'. I haven't knowingly done this, but quite often I get a sort of jealous reaction from the others. One instance, my middle son wanted football boots and my father was here. And my father said if he did some chores for him while he was here, he would give him a shilling every time he did a chore. And we told him he'd got to save up to buy his own, which I believe in. And at the same time Michael needed some more shoes and of course I went out and bought them. And when I got back with them I was told that Michael had new shoes but David had got to pay for his own. And apparently he'd told the teacher at school that he'd got to buy his own shoes – not football boots, shoes he'd said.

Girl, 3 years, profoundly deaf
Wayne will perhaps graze his knee, and he'll cry for anything, and he'll come in and he'll say 'You cuddle Jean but you don't cuddle me when I'm poorly,' and I'll say 'Come on then' and then he's all right. He can't understand that when he was Jean's age, and when she was a baby until she was about one, 'cause you cuddle babies more, don't you? And he couldn't seem to understand that he was cuddled at that age. He wanted to be cuddled as much as she was at three. He couldn't understand that when he was one he got as much cuddles as she does.

When the mothers were asked if the other children seemed jealous of the deaf child, of the 106 families with other children of an appropriate age, i.e. between 1 and 14 years of age, thirty-five (33 per cent) said there was a lot of jealousy of the deaf child, twelve (11 per cent) said there was some jealousy and fifty-nine (56 per cent) reported none at all. In the sample of cerebral palsied children[6] and normal children[7] 33 per cent of the mothers reported jealousy of the child under discussion (either a normal 4-year-old or a cerebral palsied child). Thus siblings of deaf seem to be more likely to experience jealousy than siblings of other children.

In cases where there was no jealousy, this seemed to be some times because the other children could appreciate the problems of the deaf child and the mother had taken trouble to explain.

Boy, 3 years, moderately deaf
Yes, we say to them 'You've got your hearing'.

Girl, 6 years, severely deaf
Oh yes, we've talked about it you see.

Where the children were older, often they themselves could understand and appreciate the problem, and were solicitous on behalf of the deaf child, rather than jealous of him.

Boy, 5 years, moderately deaf
No, because they're the ones that make the allowances.

Boy, 3 years, severely deaf
They understand. They've never been jealous of him, they're more protective towards him.

Girl, 6 years, severely deaf
We get feelings of strong resentment against her, but on the whole they've deep affection for her and pity for the fact that she's had to work so hard talking, and doing the things that they do normally, they've enough to understand.

Of course jealousy could operate in the opposite way – it could be the deaf child who was jealous of the other children in the family.

Boy, 5 years, severely deaf
I think he resents the freedom that the older children have. I think it's because they're older.

When mothers were asked whether their deaf child seemed jealous of other children in the family, of the 106 with siblings of an appropriate age, twenty-nine (27 per cent) showed a lot of jealousy, twenty (19 per cent) showed some jealousy, but the majority, fifty-seven (54 per cent), showed no jealousy at all.

Mothers were further asked, knowing they had a deaf child, what they felt about having more children. Having a handicapped child can conceivably influence such a decision in either direction. Some parents felt that their deaf child needed special attention and to have another child would detract from this.

Boy, 4 years, moderately deaf
We've got too many already. We don't want any more.

Girl, 2 years, severely deaf
Well my husband, he thinks because of Eileen's deafness I should spend more time with Eileen.

Girl, 6 years, moderately deaf
You couldn't say that your home with a handicapped child in it was the best place for a new baby. I wish we'd had another one, I'd have liked two. I think it would have done Carol a lot of good, but I'm not convinced in my own mind that it wouldn't have penalised the other child to some extent – because for instance – for a long time I had to take Carol about an awful lot. I had to take her to the hospital every day at one stage, well I couldn't have done that with another child without leaving the other child with somebody else all the time. I don't think this would have been quite right.

On the other hand, some parents felt that another child would help the deaf child. As many of these mothers stressed, the decision to have another child was not one to be taken lightly. Always at the the back of their mind was the feeling that this child too might be handicapped.

Girl, 5 years, severely deaf
I didn't want any more. But we realised that a baby would do her good.

Girl, 4 years, severely deaf
I wouldn't mind having another one, at least, but I think I should worry all the way through.

Girl, 4 years, moderately deaf
No, I never did want an only one, but I had a lot of doubts and worries while I was expecting the second one. I never enjoyed carrying her at all – I was bottled up and worried to death. I had visions of what else could go wrong. Having had something go wrong and not realising the possibilities I really thought about all the possibilities for a second baby – what else could go wrong. I think I was very relieved when she arrived. I had a much better time having her. I think that is why I was so elated afterwards.

Of course the critical issue is not so much whether the parents feel they would like to have more children or not, but whether having a deaf child had made them change their minds. In only just over a quarter (thirty-three, 27 per cent) of cases did it in fact make a difference, and this difference was always a decision *not* to have any more children. No parents had changed their minds about the number of children they wished to have, and decided to have more children on finding that one of their children was deaf. In the families where there was no change in attitude, sixty-four (52 per cent) intended to go on and have more children[8] and twenty-five (21 per cent) considered their families to be complete.

The great demands made on the mother by a deaf child could possibly affect the mother's health – particularly as some of the mothers felt their child's deafness cut them off to a certain extent from the world outside their family.[9]

Boy, 5 years, moderately deaf
It's made me more sort of, how can I put it, it's made me edgy. I'm always tense. I can't relax like I used to be able to relax, you know. I can't stand to hear him cry. You know, if he cries I'm there, sort of thing, I am more tense: I am very tense to what I used to be. I live on my nerves a lot more than what I used to.

Boy, 3 years, severely deaf
I'm a pretty healthy person, thank goodness. I've only been run down once, and that was this year waiting for the hearing aid. It worried me because I knew he needed it. And I did go to the doctor, but it was the first time, and I was on nerve tablets much to my disgust. I was ashamed of myself, but I needed them. I think if I hadn't gone to the doctor's, I might have broken down completely.

When the mothers were asked, 61 per cent felt themselves to be in good health, 28 per cent to be moderately healthy, 7 per cent to be in poor health and 4 per cent to be generally run down. When they were asked 'Do you find that you get run down or depressed?' Eighty-seven (71 per cent of all mothers) said they did get depressed. About four out of ten of all mothers interviewed (forty-eight) had visited their doctor because of feelings of depression. It is a pity that we have no comparison data from mothers without handicapped children. Clearly not all the depression is due to having a deaf child, as mothers of normal small children often feel run down or depressed. Until such data is available we can only speculate as to the contribution of the problems of the deaf child in the mother's feelings. Nevertheless, four out of ten mothers of deaf children does seem a high proportion, and worthy of note.

NOTES

1 The interview situation is described in Appendix III with a special discussion of the questions asked about marriage.
2 In the 122 familes: four mothers had separated from the fathers of their deaf children three of these had remarried; one father had left the mother of his deaf child, keeping the child with him; one family had broken up, the children being cared for by an aunt (who in all respects was as a mother to them); two marriages were on the verge of breaking up.
3 No questions whatsoever were asked about the parents' sex life.
4 Between 1 and 14 years.
5 S. Hewett (1970), *The Family and the Handicapped Child* (Allen & Unwin, London).
6 S. Hewett, op. cit.
7 Newson and Newson, unpublished data.
8 Or had already done so by the time of the interview.
9 These feelings of being cut off are discussed in more detail in the next chapter.

Chapter 9

The Family and the Community

It is often assumed that parents of handicapped children are less able to go out together, either because they are more reluctant to leave a handicapped child, or alternatively, because it is more difficult to get a baby-sitter for a handicapped child – a point made by one or two parents.

> Boy, 2 years, severely deaf
> We can't obtain any babysitter, because we would have to have a babysitter who knows or understands him. We can't leave him with anybody.

Overall, however, when mothers of deaf children were asked how often they did manage to leave their children and get out together with their husbands, the replies were very similar to those of parents of normal children (Table 9.1).[1]

The same sort of picture emerged when we considered whether or not the mother could leave her child during the day, if she wished to go shopping, or to the hairdresser's, for instance. As with

	Once a week or more	Once a month or more	Seldom	Once a year or less
All deaf	21% (25)	26% (32)	30% (37)	31% (38)
Deaf 3·6–4·11 years	24% (10)	21% (9)	36% (15)	19% (8)
Normal 4-year-olds	25%	16%	26%	33%

Table 9.1 Amount parents of deaf children go out in the evenings compared with parents of normal children

some mothers of normal children, for some mothers of deaf children there were acute problems of not being able to leave their child.

Boy, 4 years, profoundly deaf
No we never left him. Never left him – any time. We've tried. When I *had* to go to hospital and my husband were working that was different. When I was pregnant with Dominic you see, I had to go for check up and things like that. Me mother used to say 'Let me try this afternoon, leave him with me.' But no. He'd get that upset he'd make himself poorly over it, so I stopped leaving him altogether. In fact I started taking him with me, towards the end. I had to take him to the clinic with me.

Boy, 4 years, moderately deaf
He cries if I leave him, he still cries. If I'm upstairs and he's come in off the yard he'll cry for me.

Some mothers felt that because of the child's deafness, because of the fact they could not explain to him what was going on, that they should not leave him.

Boy, 4 years, severely deaf
I wouldn't go places and leave him. I think if he was normal, he's five, well I would, because you can explain where you're going and why you're going and that you'll be back in an hour's time. But you can't explain where you're going and why. It's explaining things again.

However, when we look at the figures we find that in practice mothers of deaf children were able to leave their child during the day as much as mothers of normal hearing children (Table 9.2).

	Can be left	Never left
All deaf	71% (86)	30% (36)
Deaf 3·5–4·11 years	67% (28)	33% (14)
Normal 4-year-olds	69%	31%

Table 9.2   The extent to which deaf and normal children can be left during the day

What about those occasions when the deaf child is to accompany the family? Does his handicap limit the social events that the family can indulge in? As far as outings and holidays were concerned, most parents felt the child's deafness had made little difference. Eighty-three per cent (101) felt they did exactly the same as they would normally have done, whereas 17 per cent (twenty-one) had made changes in their plans – not going away at all, not going such a long distance, or taking self-catering accommodation where in other circumstances they might have stayed in a hotel.

In the area of social activities, more parents felt their activities had been curtailed. Visiting friends or relations could be more difficult.

Boy, 2 years, severely deaf
We don't take David to see anybody who is civilised – that's what it boils down to. I don't like him to misbehave, and he's liable to go berserk, and they don't understand. If they have high windows and he can't see out of it, he'll climb up to see the other side, and people say 'Why don't you tell him to get down?' but we can't tell him to get down.

Boy, 4 years, severely deaf
Before we had the children we used to have a lot of family get-togethers, and we don't now, and I feel a lot of it is because of Christopher.

If there is such a problem one might expect this to have special impact on the mother. Some mothers did find social activities a problem.

Boy, 2 years, severely deaf
To some extent yes, it ties me. Because I do not take him, because he's not been a really well-behaved child, I will not take him to say, a coffee morning – something like that.

Boy, 4 years, severely deaf
I think it does. Well you see I haven't ever neighboured a good deal, but I know since I've had Christopher, whereas people would sometimes say 'Come over and have a cup of tea', once you've got a handicapped child, and they're probably not as obedient, shall we say, as a normal child, they don't ask you.

Some mothers found the noise their children made particularly embarrassing. Supermarkets or buses were places most often mentioned.

Boy, 3 years, moderately deaf
If he's in a supermarket or something with me or something, he'll go uh-uh-uh-uh-uh-uh, and everybody's sort of looking, and you feel yourself going all sort of hot and bothered. But it's not so bad now as it was initially, you know.

Boy, 5 years, moderately deaf
I think one of the worse things is if he's holding a conversation on a bus with me. I feel funny. I call it being embarrassed but the teacher told me I wasn't to be embarrassed, but I do feel funny if we're on a bus because everybody's looking at him and I know what he's on about and they haven't got a clue, you know. And that's just about the worse bit I think because in a shop you can walk in and walk out but on a bus you're stuck. And you're holding a full-scale conversation and everyone else is just looking amazed and they haven't a clue what he's saying. I feel like turning round and saying 'He's saying so-and-so, you know.' I think that's the worst bit.

Boy, 4 years, severely deaf
Sometimes when I'm out with Christopher he makes funny noises. It can be embarrassing, but he's my child, so I have to get on with it.

Deafness is such that there are no immediately obvious signs to a casual passer-by that a child is handicapped in this way, in the way that a wheelchair can indicate some physical disability, or a white stick, blindness. The only indication might be the hearing aid, though not all deaf children wear aids, and some take them off to go out (see p. 108 above). The hearing aid itself is not conspicuous, and even if observed is often taken to be a transistor radio. The lack of obvious indications of the handicap of deafness is seen as desirable by most parents who want their deaf children to be considered and treated as normally as possible. This does have disadvantages, however, in that it can result in misunderstandings of the parents by others who assume that any anti-social behaviour on the part of the child is a product of inadequate parental discipline. The trouble is that parents are not in a position to explain their problems properly to casual acquaintances who may be quick to jump to false conclusions about parental inadequacy.[2] Mothers varied in their approach, some feeling embarrassed, but that they had no alternative but to press on regardless (see last quote). Other mothers took the more defiant attitude that it was up to people in general to accept the handicapped child.

Boy, 3 years, moderately deaf
Anywhere I go, he goes.

Boy, 4 years, moderately deaf
I think people ought to accept people like Karl.

Boy, 4 years, severely deaf
I think if they are lonely it's their own fault. When I was . . .
when Stephen was a baby I felt I wanted to shut me and him
away – because I thought it was so . . . And it took me a while
to come round. Now he just goes where I go and if he meets
someone he comes along as well.

The problem can only be helped by better education of the
public into difficulties faced by the parents of normal-looking handicapped children. One obvious source of this education is the
parents of deaf children themselves. Although one may feel they
have enough to do in caring for their own deaf child, they have
the information and the contacts with all sections of the population that can ultimately expand the awareness of society as a whole
to the problems of deaf children.

The mothers were asked whether they felt that having a handicapped child cut them off from other people at all. Some mothers
expressed feelings of loneliness in that they felt different from
other mothers.

Boy, 3 years, severely deaf
I thought it at first. I'm not lonely now, but I just feel sort of
. . . when I'm with a lot of mothers with children his age that
were normal, and I felt that they didn't understand, especially
when they would make comments about his behaviour – more
so than before we found out that he was deaf than anything,
when he was a baby – I felt it much more then when he was a
baby, and other babies his age were sitting up, and walking and
feeding themselves and drinking out of cups.

Boy, 5 years, severely deaf
Well you are isolated. They are so different, you can't communicate with other mothers in the same way, and the children
can't. They're normal in the way they develop physically I suppose, but in their habits . . . You haven't got anything to talk
about when they say 'Oh she said so-and-so and so-and-so
today.' You see there's nothing.

Problems could also arise because other mothers felt embarrassed
about the deaf child.

Boy, 5 years, severely deaf
At the beginning – yes. It's not that you feel lonely, but other
people are too embarrassed to say anything.

G

However, only 8 per cent of the mothers did experience loneliness to the extent that they felt it was a problem. Some mothers in fact had found the reverse. The child's handicap opened up their social life for them – either through contacts with other parents of handicapped children, or because of the interest shown by their friends and neighbours in their child's handicap.

Girl, 4 years, profoundly deaf
In actual fact I think you make more friends with a handicapped child because everyone wants to know what it's all about. It's a great talking subject.

Boy, 2 years, severely deaf
It can make you lonely, I can quite see that it can. Certainly it can take so much of your time that you've little left for anything else. But you see in our case it actualy channelled us out into something else, in as far as we got in with this association and we got out meeting all the mothers at the school, this sort of thing, probably far more than we would have done with a normal child.

Girl, 2 years, degree of deafness not known
Well, people always seem to be stopping and talking about her, and I belong to different associations because she is handicapped, I've met a lot more mothers. Whether it gets worse as she gets older and the handicap becomes more apparent I don't know.

Boy, 5 years, moderately deaf
If anyone sees you, and he's got his hearing aid on they stop and talk to you.
(Q: Do you mind this?)
No. I only mind when they say 'What a shame.'

This last quote raises an issue which many parents who have not handicapped children themselves wonder about. With traditional English reserve, many people somehow feel that to mention or ask about a child's handicap is being nosy or intrusive. Overall, 91 per cent (111) of the mothers of deaf children welcomed people showing interest in their child. As can be seen from Table 9.3, this did not depend on whether or not they had experienced other people asking about their child. The only reservation many mothers made, as indicated in the last quote, was that although they appreciated interest shown, they did not want pity, either for themselves or for their children.

	Mother likes interest	Mother dislikes interest
Interest has been shown	45% (55)	6% (7)
No interest shown	46% (56)	3% (4)

Table 9.3   Mother's feelings about people showing interest in her deaf child related to her experience of interest shown

Boy, 4 years, moderately deaf
They say 'Oh, what a shame.'
(Q: Do you mind if they say that?)
Yes I do, because I don't think it is a shame. I think he's a little bit handicapped, he's not got as much advantage as the other children, but he's not that different.

Parents seem more likely to be hurt by the child's handicap being ignored than by people drawing attention to it.

Boy, 3 years, moderately deaf
At one time when people first realised that Nigel was deaf and noticed the hearing aid they walked on the other side of the road. They didn't know how to speak to you. You felt it then, but now Nigel's had the hearing aid for two years, everybody's more or less accepted it.

Girl, 2 years, severely deaf
No they've been the opposite really. If they've ever had to stop and have us in the house they've been over-friendly to us. They won't ask me about Tina, which is unkind really. They'll speak to you and be really kind but never will they bring up the subject about Tina being deaf. All the time you know they want to know. That is unkind as far as I'm concerned.

As already mentioned (p. 193 above) people are embarrassed with parents of handicapped children.

Girl, 6 years, severely deaf
People are embarrassed. I think they're guilty. You know they feel rotten that you've got a handicapped child and they haven't. They don't want a handicapped child but they wish you hadn't got one.

For many other people, the wish is not to pry in a way that may be hurtful to the parents of the handicapped child.

Girl, 4 years, severely deaf
They don't like to talk about it to you, I think for fear of upsetting you, but it's never worried me.

The same seems to apply when it comes to interacting with the
deaf child. Many people hold back through embarrassment, or
feelings of inadequacy.

Girl, 4 years, profoundly deaf
I have a sister, she only lives round the corner and even now
she cannot talk to Veronica without laughing. She feels silly.
You have to just put yourself out that little bit.

Boy, 5 years, profoundly deaf
They think because he can't hear, they don't have to speak to
him. I've found this in a number of people when I've gone on
the bus or anywhere. They smile but they sort of look wary of
them. I don't think they know what to say.

Girl, 3 years, severely deaf
Yes. People are very embarrassed. They don't know . . . I find
that people, they don't talk to her. Someone said to me a little
while ago, well, how do you communicate with her, and I said
'I talk to her' and they looked at me as though I were daft, you
know – what's she talking about. People are not quite sure what
to do with her. It's not that they mean to be, they don't mean
to be that way, they don't know how to go on. The truth of the
matter is that there isn't enough known about deafness. The
general public, they don't know enough about it.

This is sad because deaf children above all others would benefit
from being talked to. As the last quote says, people just do not
understand about deafness. They may show sympathy and concern,
but when one gets down to it, sympathy and concern are not
enough. Parents of deaf children feel a need for understanding of
their problems.

Many people do not see the link between deafness and learning
to talk. They can say 'I'm sorry he's deaf, why doesn't he talk', in
the same breath.

Girl, 5 years, severely deaf
They expect too much of her. They don't dream that she can't
talk.

Girl, 5 years, severely deaf
Well I don't think . . . people don't realise that deaf children

can't talk. This is the main thing – they think that they should talk. They don't realise that they can't talk, so of course it makes you embarrassed when you have to tell them she can't talk.

Boy, 3 years, severely deaf
No I don't think they're aware of all it implies. They think it's just the same as an old person, that's just gone deaf. I don't think they realise the difference between going deaf when you're old, when you've already got speech . . . you know, some friends I've got they can't seem to associate being deaf with not being able to talk even. They seem to think that speech probably isn't connected with deafness. I sometimes find myself explaining why he doesn't talk. I mean sometimes if I say 'Well he's deaf – that's why he doesn't talk,' it doesn't seem enough.

As this last mother points out, much of the difficulty is because, in general, knowledge of deafness is based on association with the elderly hard of hearing, who present a very different picture from the child who is deaf from birth. Having to speak clearly to a hard-of-hearing person is very different from trying to communicate with a child deaf from birth.

Boy, 5 years, moderately deaf
You just think deaf's deaf and that's it. You don't realise that there's a lot of different ways of being deaf and you don't just have to holler to everybody you meet that's deaf.

And then of course there is the fallacy that wearing a hearing aid puts everything right.

Boy, 5 years, moderately deaf
Most people seem to think that if they've got a hearing aid they should be normal. You know – 'If they've got a hearing aid why can't they hear you, why can't they come out and speak.' They just don't understand. It's the general feeling that if you've got a hearing aid it's like some magic box that puts everything right.

Boy, 3 years, severely deaf
I think everybody needs educating in talking to deaf people. They don't know. I didn't. I couldn't blame anybody because I hadn't an idea. I had the impression that a lot of people do, that when they have a hearing aid this is it. Everything's OK.

Girl, 6 years, severely deaf
They don't think . . . they always tend to think if a child has

a hearing aid, well that puts everything right. I don't think they understand about language and the use of language. I don't think people understand how important language is. They don't realise what a tremendous handicap it is in everything she does.

Of course, if it is difficult for people to see the communication problem that deaf children have, it will be all the more difficult for them to appreciate the associated problems linked with communication difficulties that have been described in detail in this book.

Boy, 4 years, profoundly deaf
I don't think normal people understand. They don't realise.

Boy, 2 years, severely deaf
No they haven't a clue. They don't realise.

Boy, 5 years, profoundly deaf
I don't think they do understand. They think because they're deaf they're quite normal. They don't know the frustrating times you have. A few people round here, they think – 'Oh well, Derek's deaf, you just don't speak to him.' I think they think you just let them do as they like. They don't realise the hard work you've got to put into it.

Most parents felt very much that deafness as a handicap was not understood. People may or may not be sympathetic; the majority do not understand (Table 9.4).

	Friendly	Unfriendly	Varies	Total
Aware of difficulty	21% (26)	0 (0)	6% (7)	27% (33)
Not aware of difficulty	41% (50)	11% (14)	21% (25)	73% (89)
Total	62% (76)	11% (14)	26% (32)	

Table 9.4   People's attitude to a deaf child

From the point of view of a person with little experience of communicating with the deaf, which is a large section of the population, embarking on an attempt at communicating may seem potentially dangerous. If one is not heard the first time, it may be necessary to repeat a remark over and over again. We all know how trite a casual comment can seem after three or four repetitions.

There is the problem of knowing whether to shout, talk slower, talk louder, repeat the same thing or rephrase it. All this may lead to the most well-meaning person giving up. Parents, however, wish for their deaf child to experience the many and varied contacts that the normal child makes automatically, and such contacts are essential to the development of the deaf child. Once over the initial hurdle, it is easy to talk with a deaf child, even if answers are limited, and most parents are only too keen to help in establishing such communication.[3]

Parents compared the attitude of the public toward their deaf children unfavourably with the attitude to blind children.

Boy, 3 years, severely deaf
Everybody thinks if you're blind that's disastrous, but they don't seem to think that deafness is quite the same as blindness. In actual fact it's been proved that it's worse – if you're stone deaf, that is.

Boy, 4 years, moderately deaf
It's getting through to them when they're deaf. That's only snag, isn't it? Well you see if you've got a lad what's blind he can read braille, they can be taught braille and one thing and another. A lad that's disabled he can be taught to use his hands, but when they're deaf . . .

Girl, 2 years, severely deaf
I'd like to see more lectures about it. I'd like to see films about it on television, or talks on radios. Or collections for them to give them more, like the blind; I know the blind are handicapped more than the deaf but they get twice as much money given. Nothing's for the deaf people. On the television it's 'This child's blind, watch it cross the road.' Nothing about the deaf children at all.

Boy, 6 years, severely deaf
No, really, you find deafness is a problem people don't attach very much importance to, probably because it's not a visual handicap. I don't think enough notice is taken of it. I don't think enough attention is given to the deaf at all; it is really a terrible handicap.

Girl, 3 years, severely deaf
I don't think there's much information given about deaf children, I don't. There is not as much as about blind children. Because I'll tell you for why. When it happens to us the neighbours and

friends say 'Well can't something be done? She can have an operation can't she?' They couldn't believe that there's such things, and nothing can be done and this is it. Deafness they can't . . . It's no fault of their own, as I say, there's not enough publicity – there's not.

This attitude is hardly surprising when one considers that the blind receive charitable donations to the tune of £2,000,000 a year compared to the £200,000 received for the deaf. For the general public the problems of the blind are easier to understand, and it is easier to offer tangible help.

Where does the solution lie? One can hardly blame the general public simply for being ill-informed. Some mothers appreciated that people could not necessarily be expected to understand the problems of deafness. After all, they themselves had not understood before they had a deaf child.

Boy, 3 years, moderately deaf
I don't think people know what it's like to be a mother of a deaf child – they don't know about the patience you have to have.

Girl, 3 years, moderately deaf
People don't understand. Mind you, I didn't myself until I'd got one – you know.

Boy, 4 years, severely deaf
Well you see most of them have got normal children and . . . well, I am myself, I would never ever have believed, having had three normal children, the difference a deaf child, or a handicapped child could make, and I don't think people really understand what it is like, what you're up against.

Girl, 5 years, profoundly deaf
A lot of them you see – I think you've got to be the parent of a deaf child to really understand, because I don't think anybody really understands until you live with them. I mean they can say you shouldn't do this, and you shouldn't do that but they're not living with the child.

In this context, mothers were asked whether or not they did explain to people that their child was deaf, and about the problems they had. Some mothers did make a point of explaining that their child was deaf, sometimes as a matter of principle.

Boy, 3 years, moderately deaf
No, as I say we don't make a thing out of it at all, we just accept

the fact that he is, and we tell everybody that he is, I think it's because we've told everybody right from the beginning. It hasn't come as a shock to anybody because . . . We tend to take this attitude completely.

Girl, 4 years, severely deaf
Yes, to start with. Yes, not so much adults but children. I'll say now Brenda can't hear, they don't know how to treat her but within minutes they are chatting to her.

Boy, 3 years, moderately deaf
I think it would make a mother lonely because lots of mothers are ashamed of the fact that their children are handicapped. We've never made a thing about his handicap. We've told everybody exactly what was wrong with him from a tiny child. We never hide the fact that he's handicapped in any way. If we're out and he hasn't got his hearing aid in, and somebody talks to him and he doesn't appear to take any notice, we say to them, 'Well he's not being funny, he's a bit deaf.' With a handicapped child parents tend to protect them, and by protecting them they keep away from other children and other parents, and this is why they become lonely, but I don't think you need to become lonely because you've got . . . (phone rings).

Some, as this last mother indicates, take on the somewhat more difficult task of trying to explain how a child's deafness is being reflected in his behaviour.

Girl, 2 years, severely deaf
I tend to tell people – because it always seems to me that if they talk to her and she doesn't answer – not to everybody who says 'Hello' to her, but somebody who sort of – you know if you're having a long train journey and somebody's talking to her, I think it's only fair to tell them that she's not going to answer back and talk to them, sort of thing. I think because I don't look as though 'poor child' sort of thing it doesn't embarrass them.

Girl, 4 years, severely deaf
She's getting to the stage now where you have to tell people that she's deaf, because at the time they'd say 'Hello dear, what's your name?' and she just smiled and it didn't matter when she was tiny, and children don't answer anyway. But now it looks as though she's just being rude or stupid, so I tend to say to even casual people, 'Well, Brenda's deaf, but talk to her.' I'll say 'Do

talk to her, but you must look at her.' The people I see more often, obviously you explain it further and you tend to chat about it.

Girl, 3 years, profoundly deaf
Well I used to explain a lot before she had her hearing aid, particularly on the bus. A lady would perhaps give her a sweet and she'd more or less snatch it. The lady didn't know she was deaf and it just looked as though she was ignorant. One lady did say 'She's ignorant, isn't she?' And it got me a bit . . . and I said 'What do you expect, she can't hear' oh and she went that red, she said 'Oh, I am sorry.'

As many mothers pointed out, in quite a number of situations it could be very difficult to explain; there was thus an understandable tendency only to explain if it came up.

Girl, 3 years, profoundly deaf
Well if it's a crowded bus you don't want to tell everybody, but if it does crop up in the conversation I say 'Well, you know, Denise can't hear,' and they'll say 'Oh – can't she?' But I don't go up to people and say 'She can't hear.'

Boy, 4 years, moderately deaf
I explain to close friends, but you know others, if they say 'What's wrong?' but they don't. I took him down on the bus Monday, the bus conductor tried to talk to him and he said to me 'He's shy' and I said 'Yes he's shy' and that's all I said. I mean people on the outside they, you know, you explain it and before you know anything the whole bus is talking about it.

It can be a very difficult matter to bring the subject up in casual conversation oneself. One mother explained that unless she blurted it out at the start, she found it very difficult to mention it at all later on.

Girl, 6 years, severely deaf
Well I either blurted it out right at the beginning so that they knew or I avoided it, and it just depended on my feelings at the time.

Only two mothers did *not* explain that their child was deaf as deliberate policy and perhaps it is significant that both these were immigrants.

Girl, 2 years, severely deaf
If someone doesn't know she is deaf no one can tell she is a deaf

child, no one can tell. My husband's relatives don't know she is a deaf child. Everyone speaks to her as a normal child, and in her way she tells them back what she wants and what she doesn't want. Only my Mum knows about it, that she is a deaf child. No one else knows. I don't want to tell anyone else.

Girl, 2 years, severely deaf

I would prefer English people. Indian people, they think if it's a deaf child there is something wrong with the household or something like that, and I don't like her to mix with our Indian society. I would like her to mix with English people. I have got a few Indian friends but I haven't told them she is deaf.

NOTES

1 The responses of parents of cerebral palsied children also showed a similar pattern. See S. Hewett (1970), *The Family and the Handicapped Child* (Allen & Unwin, London).

2 This is a well-known problem for the parents of autistic children; see J. and E. Newson, *What Is an Autistic Child?* (prepared for the Nottingham and District Society for Autistic Children).

3 For those who are interested to know how they can talk to deaf children, the leaflet *Points for Speakers about Deaf Children* by Gordon M. L. Smith, in its section 'When you meet a deaf child', provides an excellent guide. This leaflet is obtainable free from the National Deaf Children's Society. A recent booklet published by Action Research for the Crippled Child, *Does He Take Sugar in his Tea – How to Relate to Disabled People*, also discusses this issue, though the emphasis here is more on talking to adults who become deafened later in life.

Chapter 10

Overview

Throughout this book, we have considered the deaf child and his activities, the deaf child as a member of his family and the impact of deafness within his society. In many ways the deaf child is similar to his normal counterparts – sometimes good, sometimes naughty. He has a sense of humour, can be a source of fun and games and enjoys exploring and investigating his world.

And, also like normal children, deaf children present a diversity of personalities. There is no one typical deaf child. Some are active, some are quiet, some are friends with everyone they meet, some are shy, some are clean and neat, some are almost always dishevelled.

Boy, 3 years, severely deaf
We get lots of laughs out of him, you know. Well he's a great imitator. When he starts trying to imitate – and it's comical when he's dancing, when he tries to balance – just funny things in general

Boy, 4 years, moderately deaf
I like his ways really. His way of getting round you, and he'll come and love you in ever such a sweet way.

Boy, 3 years, partially hearing
He's company. He's full of life all the time. He always has a cheeky grin. There's always something interesting to find out with him.

Boy, 3 years, moderately deaf
He's got a tremendous sense of humour. He's a nice person, even although he's only three. You can't really not like him. He does all sorts of things and thinks they're a great joke. He'll see his

Dad coming, and he'll get his slippers and run upstairs and put them under the bed, and come down and laugh – and say 'Slippers Daddy?' – you know.

Boy, 4 years, partially hearing
We do tend to be a bit lovey-dovey with each other, you know, because we've got more time. We tend to leave the housework a bit and enjoy each other's company.

Boy, 4 years, moderately deaf
He's one hundred per cent alive is John. He's like that with anybody who sees him, he gets to know them.

But in some ways the world for the deaf child is different. What has emerged in our picture of the deaf child is that to some extent he lives in a segmented world. Continuity is lacking. Firstly it is lacking because he has not the language to communicate and this has deep implications, not only for his present behaviour but also for his understanding of events and his ability to anticipate the future. One mother described how she watched her three children preparing for Christmas – making cards, hanging up decorations and so forth. All of them were happy and excited, but whereas her two hearing daughters experienced it all as leading up to a climax on Christmas Day, her deaf daughter could not properly appreciate what was going on or anticipate how it would come to a natural end. After Christmas she was unhappy, wanted to re-wrap the presents, to continue to make cards; the structure of the whole situation had been missing for her.

Girl, 5 years, profoundly deaf
Well I find the hardest thing is when we're going out weekends, that Saturdays and Sundays is different from the week, you know. This is the hardest, you know, to say like tomorrow is Saturday and we're going out. And when she's had a holiday she doesn't realise its a holiday, and she doesn't want to go back to school. And when we go to the seaside, the only time she knows is if she sees me packing a suitcase. Other than that, she's got no idea when she's going to the seaside or anything. Where Christopher will say 'Two more weeks, Mummy, and we're going away.'

Continuity – the ability to bind events into a natural time sequence – is lacking, secondly, because the life the child lives is divided up with no connection between one situation and the next. Mummy knows little of what goes on at school, the school knows little of the day-to-day activities at home. Even the chat with

Daddy when he comes in from work drawing together the day's events cannot be as full and complete as it is with the hearing child.

Also rationality is lacking. 'Because' is a concept that is often missing altogether. Things must seem to happen because they do, and things are forbidden because they are without rhyme or reason. For the hearing child it may be 'You can't have a biscuit because we've run out.' For the deaf child it is simply 'No.'

For parents, too, many problems of bringing up their children were similar to those raised by hearing children. However, there do seem to be certain problems that parents of deaf children have beyond those of bringing up children in general. For many parents most of these problems come under the general umbrella of trying to allow and compensate for the child's handicap while not spoiling him.

In many issues this problem rears its ugly head. In order for the deaf child to learn to communicate he needs a great deal of special concentrated attention. Is it possible to give a deaf child all this attention without spoiling him? This is a problem which concerns many parents.

> Girl, 6 years, moderately deaf
> The one thing in which people could say we do spoil her, if in fact this is spoiling and here again I don't know if it is, we do give her a great deal of attention – but I don't see how you can teach a deaf child to talk without giving them endless attention. I don't know how you win over this, but it's very demanding of your attention. What can you do – they say 'Talk to them, talk to them', well you can't do that if you're not attending can you. But this is very hard – because as I say she's difficult when we've got visitors or when we go out to tea. She wants to be in all the time. One can see that some of one's friends and acquaintances don't approve at all.

One mother also described how giving her son a great deal of special attention had definitely worked as regards the improvement in his ability to communicate with her, but seemed at the same time to make him much more dependent upon her (see p. 123 above).

In the question of manners, of right and proper behaviour, parents wonder how much to make allowances for the child's inability to understand, or whether they should expect and try to enforce the standards they would expect of a hearing child. Added to this is the feeling of some parents that a deaf child needs to be *better* behaved in some respects to make up for his lacks in other spheres. Bedtime was an area of particular concern. Deaf children presented far more problems of going to bed and waking in the night than hearing children. Intuitively one can link these problems to their deafness making them feel especially cut off when it was dark. On a practical basis, however, many parents found it difficult to decide what line to take. Should they reassure the child as much as possible, or insist that he went to bed and stayed there? This is a particularly difficult decision in a society that places high value on the good child – the child who goes to bed at a 'reasonable' hour, leaving his parents to enjoy the evening together, and to have an undisturbed night.[1]

In some areas of course, there is not the choice as to whether to be lenient or not. A child must learn to keep out of danger (not touch the iron, play with power points, run on the road) and this learning if anything needs to be more emphatic with the deaf child. A deaf child cannot be reminded, or called back as he approaches danger, he has to know very definitely that he is to avoid it. Of course this meant that mothers were more protective towards their deaf child than they would need to be to a hearing child of the same age (see p. 79 above).

How to explain to a deaf child what is and is not acceptable could be difficult. Explanations were necessarily simplified, warnings limited and many of the subtleties missed out.

Girl, 2 years, profoundly deaf
I think knowing where to draw the line about the discipline side of it, and not trying to be too soft, or too hard on her, because we don't want her to go into a shell, because if she once loses using her voice it's hard for her to get it back, well we don't want to frighten her. It makes you wary of where to draw the line on discipline and other communication.

In much of the literature concerning handicapped children, the issues of overprotection and rejection are given prominence. It is important, particularly in the light of the preceding discussion, to consider carefully what we mean by these two terms – it is all too easy to dismiss a complex situation with a judgemental label.

In the context of looking after deaf children, what does over-protection or rejection mean? Is it overprotective to prevent a deaf child playing in the road when one is aware that he is in more danger than his hearing siblings? Is it rejecting to send a child to boarding school when it seems (even if, in fact, it is not the case) that only such a school is in a position to provide the best learning situation for the child? Again, it is clear that in the issues already described earlier in this chapter the balance between being fair while not spoiling or making too high a demand is difficult to establish, and parents are aware of this.

In some issues though, which we might expect to indicate over-protection if it occurred, we find that parents of deaf children are likely to behave in a similar way to parents of hearing children. They were just as likely to go out in the evening and leave the child with a babysitter, or to leave the children during the day with a friend or relation. In such matters it is clearly possible to treat the deaf child like his hearing contemporaries. In other matters it is not, and the advice to parents of deaf children to treat their child as if he were normal then seems a little glib.

In another area, too, global prescriptions seem to create problems. Most advice to parents of deaf children assumes that the ultimate aim for every deaf child is integration into the hearing community (see K. M. Williams quoted in Chapter 4 and A. H. Ling quoted in Chapter 6). Whereas few would deny the desirability of this ideal for our deaf children, one wonders about the feasibility, particularly for the more severely deaf. Even for the skilled, lip reading is hard work. When one considers the difficulties in trying to lip read described by a man such as Jack Ashley who was, at the time he became deaf, well skilled in the use of language, one starts to appreciate the problems of the severely deaf child who may not have much idea what the spoken word is all about anyway.

> The mind had to register lip patterns while working like a computer to select the correct meaning from a vast number of possibilities. Lip-reading is immensely difficult, a grossly inadequate substitute for hearing. The miracle is that with all these difficulties it works at all.[2]

A booklet published by the Royal National Institute for the Deaf explains the difficulties.

> The great drawback to lip-reading is its inexactness. A number of letters which *sound* quite different to a person who can hear, look, to a deaf person to be pronounced with almost the same movement of the lips . . . This means that almost nine out of ten words have to be guessed by even the finest lip-reader in the country.[3]

One wonders if we may be asking too much of our deaf children and their parents. Do parents in turn expect too much of their deaf children, and if so, what happens when their children fail to meet these expectations? The British Deaf and Dumb Association have been very critical of the lack of realistic advice given to parents of deaf children. They talk of:

unrealistic and over-emotional promises of full integration caused parents to entertain hopes which were all too often unfulfilled and caused disillusionment;

a total failure on the part of those responsible for the education of the deaf to publicise the standard of attainments of deaf children lead to an all too ready assumption of their satisfactory and total integration into normal society;

unrealistic and over-optimistic publicity about the deaf child is also a source of confusion to the general public and misleads them in their appreciation of the needs both of deaf children and deaf adults.[4]

Parents, in fact, had little idea what they could hope for for their child in the future, and were unsure of the place their child might take in society. Most of them assumed that integration was the ideal, and a real possibility, although some did express doubts on this issue.

Boy, 3 years, severely deaf
It raises all sorts of problems for me. I'm probably neurotic and introspective about it, but this business of right and wrong – how right is it anyway to try and fit him in with the world, you know? Why can't he just be himself and it doesn't matter if he doesn't talk. And I often wonder about the cost, to the children, of the whole business of drumming sound into them. And to me a lot of the time it's at the expense of the home and child.

Girl, 3 years, severely deaf
Father: Although the thing is I don't want Isabel to mix with just deaf children. My aim is to get her to mix with more hearing children than deaf children.
Mother: Here we differ though, don't we? We do differ on this. I feel that it is such a terrible strain on her, you know. Well, I know how I'd feel I think, I try and put myself in a position such as that and I think I personally would be happier mixing with my own kind. I feel I would be happier I'll say that. Now whether Isabel's going to feel like that I've no idea, but you say (to F) . . .
Father: I say it depends on how she's brought up. If she's always mixed with hearing children . . .

Mother: As I say this is where we really do differ.
Father: We'll have to see which way Isabel bends.

The question of integration is a complex one, and the aim of facilitating integration as far as possible a truly acceptable one. However, it would seem that parents have a right to discuss and consider this, and rather than it being implicit in all the teaching that goes on, the possibilities and problems need to be brought into the open.

Many parents of deaf children did not look too far into the future. They had little experience of the deaf and did not know quite what to expect. They had their worries of course. A major concern of most parents was whether or not the child would get married and live a normal life – and linked to this, how they would explain the 'facts of life' to their children.

Boy, 4 years, profoundly deaf
It's new now, what I'm worried about is when he gets older – the things we've got to put up with then. When he starts school – the problems we've got to face then. The way the world is today – how fast young 'uns grow up and all that. There's a lot of problems there – especially with him, not being able to explain things to him. See, you can explain things to these when they get a bit older (his two hearing sisters), the birds and the bees, things like that – but how are we going to get through to James, this is what's worrying us – you know children nowadays get married when they're fourteen and have babies when they're fifteen.

Girl, 4 years, profoundly deaf
I often worry – I think it's silly really. I try and talk myself out of it, I worry if she'll get married. I mean they do get married, don't they?

Girl, 1 year, moderately deaf
I worried in case she don't get the natural satisfactions of life, I don't mean sex, I mean going with a boy. This is what got me when I realised. She won't be able to hear anybody tell her they love her and things like that. They might tell her in their own way, but it'll be different.

And there was a general fear that their child would be left out, that he would not be able to join in activities with other people, and lead a normal social life.

Girl, 4 years, profoundly deaf
I hope that she will be able to understand and talk. People don't accept you really, if you can't, as a person.

Girl, 3 years, profoundly deaf
It's very difficult to know what it's like being deaf if you've
never been deaf. I know you shouldn't, but I feel very sorry
for her, to know what she's got to go through. She's happy
enough now, but when she gets to the age when she'll be speaking
and she'll perhaps not be able to speak properly and people will
make fun of her, and that sort of thing, and she'll perhaps feel
different to everybody else. Whereas at the moment she's too
young to understand. Sometimes I do feel very sorry for her.

But their hopes for the future were the hopes of all parents.

Girl, 6 years, severely deaf
I would hope for, I think, something that is satisfying. I think
it's a mistake to aim too high – thinking of occupations initially.
I think – I would hope – because she has a lively mind obviously,
that she wouldn't have to do something that was boring, but at
the same time it mustn't be so demanding that her deafness is a
handicap, that she sees as a handicap. But I don't think you've
got to be too concerned with money, although this matters. If
you're not earning enough money then this alters the rest of your
life. I would hope that by the time she left school she had
enough interests of her own, that she could both enjoy them with
people and without people. I would hope that she'd enjoy sport-
ing activities which she could do on her own like swimming, as
well as things that she does with other people – like tennis say.
I really would hope she'd be able to read because she enjoys
books so much and I hope she'll be able to go on enjoying books
when she needs to read them.

Girl, 6 years, moderately deaf
I'm not terribly worried about the future. She's a very independent child and I hope she'll grow up to be a very independent
person. We're not bothered about academic achievements particularly. I mean if she shows inclinations – I mean, Dr A——
said this child is university material. Well, all well and good. If
she wants to go and she's able to go, we will move heaven and
earth to see that she gets there, but I don't care about that – I
mean – excepting the fact that she's handicapped I feel I want
to get her to the stage where she can stand on her own feet and
live a normal happy useful life, that's all I want. If she's
academically inclined I shall be pleased, we shall be very pleased,
and I shall encourage her all I can, but I mean it's no good
counting on this at all, because if she's going to have a com-

munication difficulty, why, then she's not going to be able to profit from the brain power she's got.

How did mothers feel that having a deaf child was different? Some of them felt a sadness for the child himself, while others felt that they were in some way cut off from their own child.

Boy, 5 years, profoundly deaf
I used to feel that, when a child's two, and he can talk to you, you're like companions, and you're at home all day with a child and you can sort of say 'Let's have a drink now', or 'Let's do this', like I can with Pauline, but with Derek I can't. I used to say it to him but I used to think – well he is in a world of his own and I am.

Girl, 4 years, moderately deaf
Yes, when she was younger I couldn't talk to her at all. I used to think – she would be telling me things, asking me things. It was a bit lonely then.

Girl, 4 years, profoundly deaf
Nothing is particularly hard to cope with. They're all things you get used to, and you've always had. I regret . . . sometimes when I see another child her age, and Brenda is bright and I could talk to her and we could chat about things, but really I suppose that's my regret, you know, for me rather than for Brenda. It's really a selfish thing. I don't like to think about it too much. If Brenda wasn't deaf, how super, you know.

Boy, 4 years, profoundly deaf
I wonder when he will ever say to me 'Can I have . . . ?' like other children do.

Giri, 4 years, moderately deaf
Well I suppose things would have been different if she weren't like it, but I don't know how it would have changed it. At least we've got something to work for, and we just have to get on with coping with it. It's not quite like I imagined it would be – having a first baby. I'd got visions of how nice it would be, and wanting a girl, and I was going to take her shopping with me, and things like that – it hasn't worked out like I expected it to. I've got a child that I can't control at times, and gets me down, and all the little things we were going to do together didn't get done – things like that. I suppose it changes your life in that way, but our social life is the same as it would have been, I suppose. We wouldn't have gone out any more than we do.

This feeling of cut-offness from the child can apply to fathers as well as mothers, in some cases more so, because as they do not usually spend as much time with their child they do not understand him as well as their wives do.

Girl, 6 years, moderately deaf
Well, he talks to her an awful lot. In a special way because she's deaf, and he plays games with her to try and increase her vocabulary – that type of thing. He is a person that's very good at talking to small children – he loves to talk to small children. He's usually got a crowd of them round him when he's gardening or cleaning the car or anything like that. Just because I think he will talk to them, whereas the other chaps round here can't be bothered, Tom loves to talk to children, always has done, and I think in a way, this is one thing which is a disappointment to him, Carol being deaf doesn't respond as . . . he misses that. He misses the responses he would have got from a hearing child but it hasn't inhibited him.

The mothers were asked if their child's deafness had changed their lives. Fifty-six per cent (sixty-eight) felt that it had, and 44 per cent (fifty-four) felt that it had not. Some of the changes that having a deaf child can make have already been mentioned: more limited social contacts, not having more children, etc., but there were other more specific changes mentioned.

Boy, 3 years, severely deaf
It's limited where we can live for a start. We don't like A——— but we feel we have to stay here now.

Two of the families had not been able to emigrate because of the deaf child, though in another case emigration was going through satisfactorily. One mother was faced with the realisation that she could not go out to work, that no one else would look after her deaf child.

Girl, 1 year, profoundly deaf
I was obsessed that I wanted to go out to work, and I got the telephone directory and looked for . . . well I couldn't get a nursery because of the waiting lists, and registered child-minders, I couldn't really find any. And then my father says, 'You can't think of that because there's nowhere for Melanie', and then it sunk in, nobody wanted to be bothered with a deaf child really. You couldn't expect somebody to look after a deaf child. It made me face facts that I am the only one that will look after her.

Many mothers talked of more general changes, of how their child's handicap had changed their attitude to other handicapped children.

Boy, 3 years, severely deaf
Yes it's changed my life, but for the better. It's given me a lot more understanding of other people who've got children with handicaps, which I'd not got before, but until you've got a handicapped child you don't understand. You live in a perfect little world until you've got something like that.

Girl, 4 years, profoundly deaf
It's made me think more. It's made me – I don't know – more loving to other children. At one time if I'd seen a child with a hearing aid in I would have avoided it. It would have upset me that I couldn't have helped. But since I've been to that school and seen the other children I could love them all, whereas before I wouldn't have wanted to touch them. That's why I'm pleased my friends have accepted Samantha because I couldn't have accepted another child. But I could love any child now, I mean if I saw a physically handicapped child I used to dither. I hadn't the stomach to look even, but now I could.

Girl, 4 years, profoundly deaf
It's made me understand people a lot more. It's made me aware of a lot more problems in the world than . . . than I was aware of before. It's also made me a bit more sensitive and I can sort of see danger in too many places . . . I'd be happier if I didn't.

Boy, 4 years, profoundly deaf
It's made me more grown up than I was. It's changed me in a way – you know. I feel more older in myself than before I had Matthew – you know. It's a lot of responsibility.

Boy, 3 years, moderately deaf
I think it made us more tolerant. I think before we had him we didn't realise what handicapped children meant. You know, we thought – if they can't cope why don't they put him in a home, but there's a lot more to it, which we've realised.

Boy, 3 years, moderately deaf
I've realised a lot more things. Us eyes have been opened wider, and I've not taken things for granted as much.

The over-riding feeling one has when talking to mothers of deaf children is not that there is a child in the family who is a problem and constantly needs attention, for whom special plans have to be made, but that there is a child in the family who is cut off from the rest of them, with whom the mother cannot easily communicate.

Girl, 1 year, profoundly deaf
The only strain I did have was coming to face that she was deaf. I used to keep looking at Pete (her husband) and I used to sit watching the telly and I used to think 'She won't be able to hear that', hurting myself really and he'd watch me – he'd watch my face – he came to it straight away but I couldn't.

Because of this lack of contact the mothers often wonder about what the child is thinking and feeling.

Boy, 2 years, profoundly deaf
Not being able to talk – not being able to communicate. He does very well, mind you, it's just not being able to ask questions. They're not able to ask questions are they? I mean we're going out in the car and Susan will say 'What's that tractor doing in the field?' – well I often wonder what he thinks when he sees a tractor. I mean obviously he doesn't ask. I wonder if he works it out for himself or what. I mean Susan at this age used to ask questions all along, but he doesn't. I wonder if he thinks about things and wonders.

Girl, 1 year, profoundly deaf
I don't think she can understand why I dance. We turn that transistor on and we're dancing away, and I don't think she can understand what I'm doing. She'll try and join in though.

Girl, 5 years, profoundly deaf
I think sometimes if she sees something different, and she can't understand it—I think that sometimes upsets her. Because when it was snowing she couldn't understand that. Well I don't know whether it upset her, but she couldn't sort it out.

Boy, 4 years, severely deaf
I think sometimes things that he doesn't understand upset him. We try not to put him in a position that he doesn't understand, a position where he didn't know where he was, or what he was doing. I think that worries him.

Girl, 1 year, moderately deaf
Well I think what I've done with the others, but there again at the same time I keep putting myself in Kim's place. The other morning before I got up I just sat looking at her, and I thought

to myself, you know, when I'm talking to her all she's seeing is a mouth moving. She's not really hearing anything. Every time before I chastise her, that's why I always give her a threat. Before I even hit her, I sit and think how she's feeling. I've got to get into her world before I can even smack her, because every step you take it's got to be taken carefully. I keep trying to put myself in her place every time.

Girl, 4 years, moderately deaf
Because you can't put yourself in her position and know exactly what she hears and what she makes of life.

NOTES

1   See the new standard work: B. Spock (1966), *Baby and Child Care* (English edn, The New English Library, London).
    When doctors more recently have been emphasizing flexibility, confident parents haven't carried this to extremes either. They don't let a sleepy but obstinate baby refuse to be put to bed, because they know very well (mostly from their own childhood) that bedtime is bedtime, and that theories of flexibility have very little to do with the situation.
    Also E. Wright (1972), *The New Childhood* (Tandem Books, London). Make bedtime suit the requirements of your own child bearing in mind he should have an opportunity for something like eleven or twelve hours sleep. I would, however, add this: I think all children, certainly under the age of five, should have gone to bed by eight o'clock, not because there is anything magic about this hour but because it otherwise cuts down the amount of time Father and Mother have together as husband and wife – whether they want to entertain friends, sit and talk, or just watch television.
2   J. Ashley (1973), *Journey into Silence* (Bodley Head, London).
3   Royal National Institute for the Deaf publication (1965), *Conversation with the Deaf* (8th edn).
4   Report by a working party of the British Deaf and Dumb Association (now the British Deaf Association) formed to study and comment on the Lewis Report (1970), published by the BDDA, 3 Compton Street, Carlisle.

Appendix I

The Interview Schedule

University of Nottingham
Child Development Research Unit

City/County ....

Interviewer ....

Date ....

GUIDED INTERVIEW SCHEDULE
for mothers of deaf children aged 2–5 years

BACKGROUND

Child's full name ....

Present at interview? ....

Address ....

....

Date of birth .... *Sex:* *Boy/Girl*

Family size and position. (for each child in the family indicate sex and age; include foster children, marked F, and deceased children, marked D. Mark respondent*)

Name							
Sex							
Age							

Have you had any miscarriages or still births?
(Give dates with cause if mentioned)

Mother
1. Age ....

2. Are you working at the moment?   *Not working/part-time/full-time*
 If working   Occupation? ....
 (*if appropriate;*   Did you train for this?)
 Who looks after N/the children?
 Did you train for a job before you had children?
 If necessary;   What work did you do before you had children?

Father
3. Age ....

4. Precise occupation? ....
 Does he have to be away from home at all, except during the day?
 home every night/up to 2 nights away p.w./3 nights + p.w./
 normally away/separation or divorce/other
 Is he on shift work?   *Yes/No*

 If yes;   What shifts? ....

Other adults
5. Does any other adult live here now apart from your husband and
 yourself?
 Yes .... */No*

ORIENTATION
6. I wonder if first of all I can get an idea of how deaf N is. Can he
 hear anything at all?

7. Can he hear if you shout/talk normally close to him when he's
 not wearing his hearing aid?
                             shout/talk/no
 — and with his aid?   *shout/talk/no*

8. Does he take much notice of sounds? *(note any in particular)*

9. Has he been deaf since birth as far as you know?
   Yes/No ....

10. Do you know the cause of N-s deafness?

11. Can you tell me when you were first told that N might be deaf?
    (Who told you?)

12. Had you any idea before this that there was something wrong?
    If yes;   What made you think that?
        What did you do first?   *(Prompt:* Did you tell anyone else
        what you thought?   *Yes* ....*/No*.   Did you discuss
        it with your husband?   *Yes/No)*

13. When your doctor (or ....) told you about N, what
    did he actually say to you?

14. Did you take it in then?
    — and your husband (did he take it in?)

15. How do you feel about the way you were told?

16. What do you think is the best time to be told this sort of thing?

17. Have you been told how deaf he is?

    if yes;   Do you know the result of his last hearing test?

18. About how many hearing tests has he had?

19. Do you know if his hearing has got better or worse?
    better/worse/same/D.K./N.A.   *(ask permission to obtain audio-
                                gram if this would be useful)*

20. Has he ever been asked to do an intelligence test?
    Yes/No/D.K.

    If yes;   Who did it?
        Where was it done?
        How old was he then?
        Do you know what the result was?

21. Is N usually a healthy child?

22. Has he any handicaps other than deafness?

INDEPENDENCE

I wonder if now we can talk more generally about N, the sorts of things he does.

23. *EITHER*   Does he usually dress himself in the morning?
                 Do you give him any help with that?
                 Mother helps a lot/some help/no help given
    OR   How far can N look after himself? Can he put any
                 of his clothes on without help? *Yes/No*

                 If yes;   Which?

24. *EITHER*   Does he undress himself at night?
                 Mother helps a lot/some help/no help given.
    OR   Can he take any of his clothes off? *Yes/No*

                 If yes;   Which?

25. *EITHER*   Does he tidy up his clothes when he's taken them off?
                 Mother helps a lot/some help/no help given.
    OR   *Omit...............*

26. *EITHER*   When he goes to the toilet, does he look after himself,
                 or do you help him?
                 (*Prompt;* Does he wipe himself, or do you do that for
                 him?)
                 Mother helps a lot/some help/no help given.
    OR   Does N use a potty or the toilet yet?
                 nappies/potty/toilet

                 How much help does he need when he uses his potty/
                 goes to the toilet?
                 Mother helps a lot/some help/no help given.

27. *EITHER*   What about clearing up things he's been playing with?
                 Does he do that at all?
                 Mother helps a lot/some help/no help given.
                 If clears up: How do you persuade him to clear up his
                 things?
    OR   *Omit...............*

28. What do you feel about making a child do things for himself at this age? Do you think he should be made to do things for himself, even if he doesn't want to?

29. *If 'no' help checked 3 or more times*
    Have you taken a lot of trouble to get N to do things for himself?

Otherwise Would you like N to be doing more things for himself at this age? (*Prompt if necessary.* Does he do as much as you think he ought to be doing now?)

> *If no:* Do you think you should be stricter than you are over this or are you quite happy to leave it for the moment?

PLAY

General

30. Now what about the things he likes doing.
   What does he like doing best?

31. What toys seem to give him the most pleasure?
   Does he have firm favourites, or just play with anything he happens to pick up?

32. What about playing in the house—does he like to play on his own?
   mostly / sometimes / not at all

33. How long will he play by himself without wanting your attention?
   up to 30 mins / 31–60 min / longer

34. Does he like to be able to see you, or doesn't he mind?

35. If he keeps wanting you to do things for him when you are busy, what do you do?

36. Does he ever come clinging around your skirts and wanting to be babied a bit?
   often / sometimes / never
   What do you do? *or* What would you do if he did at this age?

37. Do you think he should be able to amuse himself most of the time, or would you expect to spend a lot of time keeping him happy
   (*explain if necessary;* when he's on his own, without other children)

38. Does he make a fuss when he has to stop playing?
   (*If necessary prompt:* When it's time for a meal and he wants to finish something he has started, what happens then?)
   fuss / a little fuss / no fuss
   If any fuss: What do you do when he does?

39. Is there any sort of play you don't allow? For instance, do you let him make a lot of noise about the house if he wants to? *yes/usually/sometimes/never*
    If usually, sometimes, never: How do you get him to be quiet when you want him to?

40. Do you let him jump on his bed and use the furniture for his play—like making a train out of chairs?
    Bed: Yes/No   Chairs: Yes/No
    Others: ..../No ....

41. Do you let him make a mess playing with water, or paint, or earth, or flour?   *Yes/No*
    Does it bother you if he gets really dirty while he's playing? *Yes/No*
    If yes; What do you do to get him to keep clean?

42. When he's playing at something, do you ever join in? *Yes/No*
    If yes; What sort of game?
    Are there any special games he likes to play with you?

43. Does he like looking at books?
    If at all; What sort of books does he like?
    Has he any books of his own?
    Do you look at books with him?
    If Yes;   How often?   *Daily/2 or 3 times p.w./ less*

44. Does he like watching television?   *Yes/No*
    If yes; What programme does he like?
    Are there any he watches regularly?

45. Have you any pets?   *Yes* ..../*No* ....
    If yes; How does N get on with......................

IMAGINATION AND FANTASY

46. Is there anything N is afraid of? (*prompt if necessary:* the way some children are afraid of tiny insects or of the plughole)
    If yes: What?
    Do you know why he is afraid of that?
    Do you know how it started?

47. Children this age often have imaginary friends; does N have any imaginary people or places he brings into his play?
    Yes/No

    If yes: How did you find out?

    What do you feel about this?

48. Does N ever pretend to do things or play at doing grown-up things?
    (*Prompt:*   play making tea, play part of mother, or doctor or something like that)
    Does he ever play with dolls?   *Yes/No*
    If yes: What sort of games?

49. Does he play these sorts of games (*such as; . . . state any mentioned*) with other children at all?

SOCIAL PLAY

50. How much does N play with other children?
    (*Prompt if necessary:* With his brother/sister? . . . with other children?)
    Siblings   *often/sometimes/never*
    Others   *often/sometimes/never*

    If never plays with other children
    Sometimes there's a problem for a deaf child – that other children leave them out. How does N feel about other children – does he he seem to want to join in?
    Yes/No

    If no: Does he respond to other children at all?

    If does play with other children

    Sometimes there's a problem for a deaf child – that other children leave them out of their games – does this happen to N at all
    Yes/No

    If yes: And does he seem to want to join in?

51. *Only if older sibs.*
    Does/do the other child/children bring their friends home to play?
    Yes/No

    If yes: Do they take an interest in N? Do they talk to him?
    Yes/No
    Do they include N in their games at all?   *Yes/No*

    If yes: What sort of games?

When (.........*sibs' names*) go out to play in the street or park, do they ever take N with them?
often/sometimes/never

52. Does he make himself understood with other children alright?

53. Does he stand up for himself, or does he let other children boss him around?

54. Will he share his toys with other children?

55. Does he understand about taking turns? (with a special toy, on swings etc.)

56. Does he enjoy a competitive game with other children – the sort of game where somebody wins?

Aggression in Play
57. What do you do if there's a disagreement or quarrel?

58. In general do you find it possible to leave N to settle his own differences at this age? (*Explain if necessary* – so long as there is no real bullying going on)

59. *If N plays with siblings*
There seem to be two sorts of disagreement he might get into – either with his brother/sister or with other children. Do you find you act differently in these two situations?
Yes/No
(Specify)

60. Suppose N comes running to you because he's been upset by another child. What do you do? *OR* What would you do if he did?

61. Do you ever encourage N to hit another child back?   *Yes/No*

If yes: Can you give me an example of when you might do that?
If no: Is there any situation in which you might do that?
(Example in either case)

Rating   encouragement of aggression in self defence/general encouragement/special circumstances/never

MEALTIMES

62. I'd like to know something about N's mealtimes now. Is he a good eater or do you have any trouble with that?
Good/varies/finicky

63. Do you have any rules about eating up food?
    Prompt as necessary:
    Are there any foods that he never has, just because he dislikes
    them?
    Yes/No
    Do you let him leave food on his plate?   *Yes/No*
    Do you let *him* decide how much he will have of a food he
    dislikes?   *Yes/No*
    If he really refused to eat something what would you do?

    Prompt all mothers: If he didn't like a meal after you'd cooked
                          it, would you make him something else?
    Yes/No

    *Rating   Unlimited pressure to finish/child normally has to eat
    meals prepared/has to eat amount he takes himself/may
    leave a little/no pressure/alternative provided after
    refusal/other.*

64. Do you mind what order he eats things in? For instance, does
    he have to eat bread and butter before he has any cake and that
    sort of thing?
    Strict on order/some attempt but flexible/doesn't mind
    Do you let him use a spoon instead of a knife and fork if he
    wants to? (*Prompt if necessary:* Would you let him if he did
    want to?)
    No/discourages/allows
    Do you let him use his fingers? (*Explain if necessary:* for things
    like pieces of meat, cut up vegetables and so on)
    Never/discourages/allows
    Do you let him get up from the table during a meal?
    often/sometimes/never/special circumstances only ....
    Is he allowed to bring toys or a book to the table?
    never/discourages/allows
    Do you have other rules about meal times (like not starting before
    everyone is served or anything like that?)
    Yes ....*/No*

65. Do you take a lot of trouble to get him to eat nicely and have
    good table manners or are you leaving it for the moment?
    much trouble/some trouble/leaving it

66. Does he make a lot of noise when he eats – this often does seem
    to be a problem with deaf children?
        Yes/No

    If yes: Do you feel there is anything you can do about it at this
              age?

H

If no: Have you taken trouble to teach him not to? (*If yes, probe* How?)

67. In general, would you say you mind very much whether a child has good table manners at this age?
    Yes/No

PERSONAL HABITS

68. Going on from table manners now, what about other sorts of habits? Has N any other little habits you've noticed? Does he twist his hair or pull his ears or anything like that?
    hair twisting .... *ear pulling* .... *thumb sucking* ....
    nail biting .... *nose picking* .... *rocking* .... *head banging* .... *dummy* .... *other* ....

69. Does he play with his private parts at all?   *Yes/No*

    If no: What would you do if he did?—Would you mind him doing that at this age?

70. Is there anything else you can think of that he does as a habit-Anything he does when he's over tired, or worried, perhaps?
    If not already mentioned – Prompt   head banging ....
                                           flapping hands ....

71. Do you try and stop him (*prompt for each one mentioned*) or don't you really mind?
    If yes: How do you try to stop him?

BEDTIME

72. Now what about bedtime?   Can you tell me what time he got into bed last night?
    Is that the time he usually goes to bed or does it vary a lot?

73. Does he have to be in bed by any special time?
    Yes ....*/No*

    If yes: If he didn't seem tired and wanted to stay up a bit longer, would you let him?
    Rating   *Rigid/flexibly rigid/flexible/no rules*

74. Does N sleep in a room on his own, or is he with somebody else?
    Alone/with .... *Same bed?* ....

75. Can you tell me exactly what happens from the time you start getting him ready for bed to the time he goes to sleep? Tell me about a typical bedtime. (*Prompt if necessary:* What's the first thing you do?)

76. Does your husband (or anyone else) help with getting him to bed? .... *usually takes full responsibility*/................. *often helps*/*mother alone*

77. Is there anything he takes into bed with him, like a teddy, or a piece of cloth, or a bottle or dummy, or anything like that? (*Prompt all*)
    soft toy/*bottle*/*dummy*/*other* ....
    Would he make a fuss if you couldn't find it one night? *Yes*/*No*

    If toy: Does it have to be that particular toy? *Yes*/*No*
    Does N ever have a bottle to go to bed with? *Yes*/*No*

    If No: Can you tell me when he gave that up for good?

78. *If not already mentioned:* Does he ever suck a dummy nowadays? *Yes*/*No*

79. Is there anything special that you always have to do at bedtime – any little game you always have, or something like that? (*Specify*)

80. Once N gets into bed, is he allowed to get out again, and play around the bedroom? *Yes*/*No*

81. Does he have the light on in his room for a while? *No light*/*night light*/*indirect*/*full light for a short time*

    If full light: Is he allowed to play with toys or books in bed? *Yes*/*No*

    If not full light: Would you allow him to have the light on and play with toys or books in bed if he wanted to? *Yes*/*No*

82. Does he have anything to eat in bed? ..../*No*
    or drink? ..../*No*
    What about sweets in bed? ..../*No*

83. What happens if he gets up and tries to come back into the room where you are? Do you ever let him stay if doesn't seem sleepy? *often*/*occasionally*/*only in emergency*/*never*

84. Suppose he was hungry about an hour after he'd gone to bed? Would you let him eat at that time?
Yes/No/Only ....

85. Do not prompt but record if mentioned spontaneously
.... *stories told or read* .... *Songs*
.... *Prayers with child* .... *Cuddling or kissing*

86. Do you have trouble in getting him to sleep? *Yes/No*
If yes: How do you cope with this?

87. Does N usually sleep right through the night? (*Exclude illness if mentioned*) *wakes often/sometimes/seldom or never*

88. Who usually gets up in the night if he wakes?

89. Do you lift him for the potty at all? *Yes/sometimes/no*

90. If he wakes (apart from needing the toilet or his potty) what does he do? Does he cry?
Lies awake quietly/tries to call parents/cries/very distressed/ seems frightened/angry/gets into parents bed as routine/other
....

If at all distressed: What seems to be the matter?
What do you do if he wakes up? (*Note any different responses for different behaviour*)

(*If the following have not been mentioned, ask*)
What would you do if he seemed frightened?

If he was just feeling sociable?

If he wanted to come into your bed?

If the following remedies have not been mentioned
Would you *ever*   let him come into your bed?
yes/no – disapprove/no – prefer other methods
get into bed with him?
yes/no – disapprove/no – prefer other methods
/N sleeps with .... */N in cot*
sit with him?
yes/no – disapprove/no – prefer other methods
get him something to eat in the night?
yes/no – disapprove/no – prefer other methods

91. *If appropriate*
Do you think the fact he can't hear has anything to do with his waking up/not settling down to sleep?
Has the doctor suggested any way of dealing with this problem?

TOILET TRAINING

92. You said that you lift/don't lift N for the potty/toilet at night.
I expect he still wets the bed sometimes doesn't he?   *Yes/No*
OR   I expect N still wears nappies at night?   *Yes/No*

   If no: Does he still wet the bed sometimes?

   If yes: How often do you find the nappy wet in the morning?

93. *If any wetting:* About how often does it happen?
   most nights/1–3 nights p.w./less than once p.w./almost never
   What do you do if you find he's wet the bed?

   A. *very concerned/mildly concerned/unconcerned*
   B. *punitive/reproachful/neutral or sympathetic*

   If no wetting: Did you have a problem over getting him dry at
                     night
                     Did you have any special method?
   Punishment/reproach/rewards/no pressure

94. *EITHER* What about in the daytime? Does he still have
             accidents sometimes?
             yes/no

   If yes: Is it mainly wetting his pants or does he dirty
              them?

   What do you do?

   If punishment not mentioned: Do you ever
   punish him for wetting/dirtying his pants?

   A. *very concerned/mildly concerned/unconcerned*
   B. *punitive/reproachful/rewarding/neutral or sympathetic*

   How did you teach him/are you teaching him to use his potty/
   the toilet?

   If appropriate: How does he let you know when he wants to use
                      the toilet?
   OR   What about in the day time – does he use his potty?

      If yes: I expect he still has accidents sometimes doesn't he?
                 Yes/No

         If yes: Is this mainly wetting his pants or does he
                    dirty them?

         What do you do?

If punishment not mentioned: Do you ever punish him for wetting/dirtying his pants?

A. *very concerned/mildly concerned/unconcerned*
B. *punitive/reproachful/rewarding/neutral or sympathetic*
How did you teach him/are you teaching him to use his potty?

(*If appropriate:* How does he let you know he wants to use his potty?)

If no: When do you think he'll be ready to use it?

GENERAL MANAGEMENT AND DISCIPLINE

95. I wonder if you could tell me now about how you and N get on together. What sort of things do you specially enjoy about him?

96. Do you show your affection towards each other quite a lot, or are you fairly reserved with each other? (*Prompt if necessary:* Do you think kissing and cuddling should be discouraged at this age?) (*Child caressed during interview? Yes/No*)

   Rating   very warm and demonstrative/warm/rather cool/negative

97. What about disagreements?   What sort of things make you get on each other's nerves?

98. Of course this is an age when children are often awkward about doing the things you ask them to, or want them to. What do you do when this happens?
   (*Dangerous situations discounted*)

99. Does he obey you fairly quickly or do you have to keep on at him to get him to do things?

   If he refuses to do something he really must do, what happens then?
   (*If M says 'I make him', prompt:* How?)

100. Do you ever promise him something in advance, as a reward for being good, or can't he understand yet about things that will happen later?
   Does/Does not

   If Does: How do you get that idea over to him?
   (*Example*)

If Does not: Is that because he wouldn't understand or because you don't believe in it?

101. Of course there are lots of things that children have to be taught at this age, and I expect some things are particularly difficult because N is deaf. What has been the hardest thing to teach N?

102. How did you teach him not to be destructive around the house, not to write on walls, or tear books?   (*Prompt:*   How did you manage this?)

103. Do you remember how you taught him to stay away from things that could harm him, a hot stove, or iron, or electricity points?

104. If you needed to stop him doing something, is there any way you can get his attention without actually going over to him?

    If yes: How?

105. Does he understand that he musn't run onto the road?

    If yes: Is there any time when you let him go out on his own?

106. Does N ever have a real temper trantrum?   *Yes/No*

    If yes: What does he do?

        How often does it happen?
        *more than one a day/most days/2 or 3 times a week/
        once a week/once in 2 or 3 weeks/once a month/less*

        What sort of thing starts them off?

        How do you deal with it?
        Do you think he ever has a tantrum because he can't
        make himself understood?

107. Does N ever try to smack you or hurt you in any way?   *Yes/No*
    What do you do?   *OR* What would you do if he did?

108. How do you feel about smacking – do you think it's necessary to smack most children?

109. Do you feel differently about smacking N at all?
    (Some people say that a deaf child needs more smacking than a hearing child, and others say you should try not to smack a deaf child. What do you feel about this?)

110. *If smacks at all:*   Do you have to be angry when you smack N
                          or do you do it simply as a punishment?

What sort of naughtiness do you smack him for?

111. Do you think smacking does him any good?   *Yes/No*

     If yes: In what way?

     Rating   A.   *Smacks only when calm/only in anger/both*
     　　　　 B.   *Believes in smacking/Believes in smacking but not deaf children/disapproves on principle/disapproves on principle but deafness necessitates.*

112. Is there anything else you do when he's naughty?
     Do you ever send him to bed?   *Yes/No*
     Do you ever send him out of a room
     or make him stay in a room as a punishment?   *Yes/No*
     Do you ever make him sit still in one place?   *Yes/No*
     Do you ever show you disapprove by deliberately
     turning your face away from him?   *Yes/No*
     Would you stop him having something he likes,
     like sweets or television, as a punishment?   *Yes/No*

113. Parents of children this age often say that they threaten punishments but don't actually carry them out. Do you find you can do this with N?   *Yes/No*

     If yes: How?

114. *If other sibs:*   Do you think you make allowances for N more than the other children?
     Yes/No

     If yes: Do they understand that this can't be helped or do they think he gets away with things, and this is not fair?

115. *If other sibs:*
     I think where there is a handicapped child the other children often do feel a bit left out. Do the other children ever seem jealous of N for the attention he gets?
     Yes/No

     If yes: What do you do about this problem?

116. *If other sibs:*   Does he ever seem jealous of them?   *Yes/No*

     　　　　 If yes: *What does he do when he's feeling jealous?*
     　　　　　　　　 How do you deal with it?

117. Is N a happy child or is he miserable a lot of the time?

What things let you know if he is especially happy or especially miserable?

118. Is there anything in particular which seems to upset or worry N? *Yes/No*

If yes: How do you cope with this? Do you try to avoid upsetting him as much as possible, or do you find it easier to let him get upset and calm him down afterwards?

119. On the whole are you happy about the way you handle N's behaviour or do you sometimes find yourself doing things you don't really approve of?

120. In general, compared with other people, do you think of yourself as being very strict, or rather strict, or rather easy going, or very easy going?
very strict / rather strict / rather easy / very easy

121. Do you agree with your husband about discipline, or is he a lot more strict or less strict than you are with children?
            more strict / same / less strict
and with N?   *more strict / same / less strict*

CONTACT WITH FATHER

122. How much does your husband have to do with N? Does he play with him a lot?
often / sometimes / never
Does he: Bath him?   *often / sometimes / never*
           Dress or undress him?   *often / sometimes / never*
           Read to him, or show him
           a picture book?   *often / sometimes / never*
           Look after him when
           you're out?   *often / sometimes / never*

If never to any of these: Is that because he doesn't want to, or because you don't want him to?

123. Does N's Daddy ever take him out on his own? How often?
Rating Twice a week / once p.w. / once p. month / rarely / never
What sort of things would they do?

124. Does he look after the other children a lot?

125. Is there anything he won't do – that he draws the line at?
N ....
other children ....

126. What about bringing N up generally – What sort of things do you and your husband feel differently about?

127. Can you tell me now about communication between N and you – how does he tell you things or explain things to you?

128. And what do you do when you want to tell him something or explain something?

    If gestures or signs mentioned
    Are there any other gestures or signs you use (besides ....)?

    If gestures or signs not mentioned
    Do you ever find yourself in situations where you have to use gestures or signs?

129. What do you feel about him using gestures at this age?

    If not mentioned: Do you think that there is any danger that it might upset his relationship with other people in any way?

130. *EITHER*
    Can he understand what you say to him at all? (*Prompt:* What sort of things?)
    OR
    You've said he understands when you say .... Are there any other words he usually understands?

131. Do you find yourself talking to him although he can't hear you? (*Prompt:* Do you sometimes read books out loud with him?)

    If yes: Do you ever do this deliberately?

132. What about singing songs or nursery rhymes?

    Does his Daddy do this at all?

    If songs or nursery rhymes: Does he enjoy you saying things to him, or singing to him?

133. Can he understand other people at all?
    (*Specify*)

134. Does he try to lip read? *Yes/No*

135. *If yes:* Do you try to teach him?

    If no: Do you feel he isn't ready for that yet, or does it seem best to leave it?

136. Can he say any words that you understand, yet?   *Yes/No*

   If yes: What sort of words?

   Does he speak in sentences at all?   *(example)*

   Is he pleased when you understand, or does
   he take it for granted?

137. Does his Daddy understand him as well as you do?
   Daddy – Better/Same/Less well

138. What about his brother/sister – can he let them know what he
   wants?

139. Could he go and fetch them/his Daddy for you?   *Yes/No*

140. Do you think other people could understand him?

141. Will he start a conversation with somebody he doesn't know very
   well?

GUIDANCE

General

142. Are there particular things that you and your husband do with
   N because he is deaf?

143. Have you had any help, or suggestions as to special things to do
   with N?   *Yes/No*

   If Yes: (a) Who from?
   How often do you see him?
   How long have you been seeing him for?

   (b) What sort of things do you talk about with him?
   How do you get on with him?

   (c) What things has he suggested that you do?
   Did he say why you should. . . .

   (d) Do you find N will let you teach him?
   (*Prompt:*   or is it more difficult because he knows
   you so well?)

   (f) Do you think the advice you have had has been
   sensible advice? Do you ever find it not very
   practical?   *(Specify)*

144. Have you seen anyone else apart from .... about N's
   deafness?

145. Has the doctor, or anyone else, taken a lot of trouble to explain N's difficulties to you?

146. Do you feel you understand his handicap as well as you want to, or would you be glad to have it explained more fully?

147. After you knew what was wrong with N, did you try and find out more about deaf children?

Have you seen any of the booklets published
by the NDCS?   *Yes/No*
Have you read any other books about the
subject, or articles in magazines?   *Yes/No*
Have you heard any talks on the radio or
television?   *Yes/No*

    If Yes: Were .... easy
                to understand?
                Were they helpful at all?
                Is there any way in which they might have been more help?
                Have you had the chance to go on any courses for parents of deaf children?

148. Do you know any mothers of other deaf children?

    If Yes: And do you find this helpful?

149. Do you think the parents of deaf children this age do need some sort of help, or isn't it important yet?

EQUIPMENT

150. What about equipment – do you know what sort of hearing aid N has?

151. Is it bought or borrowed?   *bought/borrowed*
    If borrowed: Who is lending it to you?

152. Have you found the hearing aid a lot of help to N?
    help/not help/other ....

153. How old was he when he started wearing it? ....

154. Some children don't like things in their ears, and hearing aids get in the way of play – does N mind wearing it? *Yes/No*
    If No: Did you have trouble getting him to wear it at first?

If Yes: Do you do anything to persuade him to wear it?
How much will he wear it?

155. Do you find it difficult to keep it in working order?
Yes/No/Some difficulty

156. Do you find it difficult to get spare batteries or leads?
Yes/No/Some difficulty

157. Did you have a lot of trouble getting the hearing aid?
Yes/No/Some difficulty

158. How long was it between the time it was ordered and the time
you got it?

159. Have you had any advice about using it?

160. Is there any other equipment you have, or have had?
(Specify)

Is it bought or borrowed?   *bought/borrowed*
If borrowed: Who is lending it to you?

161. Who suggested you should have this?

162. Do you find it helpful to N?

163. Have you had any help in its use?

164. Is there anything you would like, but haven't got?

SCHOOL

165. Does N go to school at all? *OR* You've said N goes/doesn't
go to school

If not at school
a) Do you know which school he will go to?
When?
b) Would you like him to go to school now?

If at school
a) Which school?

If day school
How often does he go to school?
For how long does he go?
How does he get to school?

If taxi: Does anybody go with him?
Does he seem happy to go in the taxi?
What time does he leave for school – and get home?

> *If appropriate:* Do you feel this is a long day for a child of this age or does he seem to manage all right?
>
> Do you worry about this, or do you think it's important he should get this extra start because he is deaf?

If boarding

What do you feel about him having to go away to school at this age?
Did he take long to settle?
How often do you see him?

166. a) Is this the school you want him to go to?
     Prompt: Would you prefer him to go to a day/boarding school?

   If appropriate: Why?

   b) Is the school helping N?
      If yes: In what ways?

   c) Does he like school?
      Did he like it at first?

   d) Can you go to the school and talk to them about N whenever you like?
      Prompt: Do you feel parents are welcome in the school?
      Have you had a chance to discuss him with the teachers as much as you want to?

   e) Does the school give you suggestions as to things to do at home with N?
      Do you find it possible to do these?

167. Once N starts school/Now that N has started school would you like someone to visit/continue to visit you – someone who could talk about any problems that might arise; or don't you feel that will be necessary?

CONTACT WITH OTHER PEOPLE

168. Some people say that having a handicapped child makes a mother very lonely. Do you think this is true from your experience?

169. Do you take N with you to visit friends and relations very often?
     Do they come and see you?

170. How does he get on with his grandparents – often they seem to have difficulty with a deaf grandchild?

171. *If person other than grandparents living in house*
How does he get on with .... ?

172. It seems that quite a lot of people are embarrassed with a child who is deaf – they don't know quite what to do. Do you find this at all?
(*if necessary, prompt:* Do you find that people are reluctant to play or try and talk to him – a bit shy of him?)

173. Have you ever tried to explain to friends and neighbours about N's deafness, to get them to talk to him and be generally friendly?

174. In general would you say that people are aware of the difficulties of children who are deaf?

175. How does N get on with people he doesn't really know?
Does he try to show them things and get them to play or is he shy?

176. Is he ever upset by them?

177. Do you feel your relations or friends treat him differently from your other children   (*Prompt:* Do they ever take him on outings or have him to stay?)

178. What about taking him out yourself – do you take him to the park, or when you go shopping?

179. Do you find other mothers stop and talk to you about N, because they see he is deaf?

180. Do you/would you mind this?

181. Deaf children make odd noises sometimes, don't they? Has there ever been an embarrassing moment when you've been out with N?

182. What about when you go on holidays or outings – are there particular problems with these?

183. Do you feel there are some places you just can't take him?

184. Has there ever been a time when it seemed to you that someone was unnecessarily unkind because of N's deafness (either to you or him)?

BABY-SITTING

185. Do you and your husband ever manage to leave N/the children
    so you can both go out together?
    1+ p.w./1 p.w./1+ p.m./1 p.m./ seldom/1 or less per annum

186. *If yes:* What happens when you do that? (*Prompt:* Does some-
    body come in?
    Do you pay her?)
    Paid baby sitter/Unpaid ..../*neighbour listens/*
    other children responsible/nobody

187. Do you get out without your husband?
    Does he go out without you?

188. Do you ever leave N at someone else's house for a little while?
    Yes/No

    If yes: Does he mind you leaving him? *Yes/No*

        If yes: What do you do about that?

        If No: Was there ever a time when he minded?
        (Age ....)
        What did you do?

189. Do you try to let N know when you're going out, or do you find
    it easiest to slip off without him knowing?
    (Is he usually asleep when you go out?)

190. Does it make a difference if he is with the other children when you
    leave him?
    Yes/No/No other children

191. Where would you leave him if you had to go away – into hospital,
    or something like that?

192. Would you be reasonably happy about that arrangement?

SEPARATION

193. Has N ever been separated from you for more than a day or two
    (apart from school)?
    Has he been in hospital for instance, or have you been in hospital
    since he was born?

    Details: When?
    How long?
    Visiting?

194. Would you say N behaved differently when he came home again
    – was he upset at all?

195. Talking generally now – what do you feel is N's greatest difficulty
    from his point of view?

196. And from your point of view – what is it about him you find most
    difficult to cope with?

197. At the moment, who do you rely on most for help?
    If husband – and who after him?

198. Do you feel that N's handicap has changed your life?
    (*If yes: Prompt:*   In what way?)

199. Some people say that having a handicapped child brings the hus-
    band and wife closer together, and some that it puts a strain on
    a marriage. What do you feel about this?
    (*Prompt opposite*)

200. Has your own health been fairly good since N was born?

201. Do you find that you get run down or depressed?   *Yes/No*
    If yes: Is your doctor giving you anything for that?
        sleeping tablets / tranquillisers / tonic / other

202. Do you think having N (has) changed your feelings in any way
    about having more children?

203. Have you discussed this with anybody else? (*Prompt:*   Your
    husband?)

204. Have you any suggestions to make that might be helpful to other
    mothers of deaf children? (*Prompt if necessary:*   either practical
    suggestions for looking after them or on how you managed to
    come to terms with it?)

205. What about the future – have you any particular worries?

206. What do you hope for – for N in the future?

To be completed after the interview

   Child   *Comprehension*

           Expression

           Language or gestures used during interview

           Attitude to interviewer

Housing   *Modern detached/modern semi/Victorian detached/Victorian semi/terraced with bays/terraced without bays/S.C. flat .... floor/rooms .... floor/council house on estate /council house not estate/council flat .... floor/ other ....*

Permission to obtain audiogram   *Yes/No*

Appendix II

The Interview Situation: Advantages and Disadvantages

The situation used to obtain the information provided in this book was that of the guided interview. This is described in detail by Newson and Newson,[1] but essentially it consists of a basic set of questions, in a standard form; but allows the interviewees to reply freely and not conform to set categories. The interviewer is at liberty to probe matters in depth as she sees fit.

The interviews were tape recorded, with of course the mothers' permission, though no one did in fact refuse. From these recordings, quotes were taken and items coded as relevant.

In such a situation it is always difficult to know whether what is said is an accurate representation of the situation. To facilitate the mothers' feeling free to talk, it was made clear that the interviewer was not connected with any official educational or health body, and was in no position to make reports or recommendations. Certainly it was felt by the interviewer that mothers had been straightforward with her. Many mothers did in fact say during the interview that they did feel free to talk (see p. 164 above).

Questions must be phrased very carefully to give people the freedom to give an honest answer without leading them. As illustration, the questions asked about the effect of the child's deafness on the parents' marriage will be considered in detail.

It was felt important to establish whether having a deaf child affected a marriage. Obviously this is a very sensitive area, and very difficult to probe. Questions about marriage were asked late on in the interview schedule. The form of the question needs some discussion. The question was:

Some people say that having a handicapped child brings the husband and wife closer together, and some that it puts a strain on a marriage. What do you feel about this?

If the reply was to the effect that they had been brought closer together, then a prompt question was used:

Has there ever been a time when it (or N being deaf) has been a strain?

and similarly, if the reply to the original question was to the effect that it had been a strain for the couple concerned, then the prompt question used was:

Has there ever been a time when it (or N being deaf) has brought you closer together?

If the reply was to the effect that it had made no difference, a further probe was made:

Has there ever been a time when it (or N's deafness) has brought you closer together, or been a strain?

Again prompts were used if appropriate:

and has it ever been a strain?
and has it ever brought you closer?

It will be noticed that the question suggests that people have found having a deaf child a strain, i.e. that this is a legitimate answer to this question, and they are further given a second opportunity to mention problems if they have occurred. The assumption is that parents will be reluctant to say that having a deaf child has made a difference if it has not, and thus it is legitimate to probe the possibility of it having made a difference as far as possible.

The question also allowed the mother a possibility of opting out answering it as a personal question. As it ended

What do you feel about that?

she could give a very general, non-personal answer. Only one or two mothers did this; in these cases the answers were not followed up further.

In general terms, one or two questions employed the phrase 'Some people say . . . and others say . . .', apart from the question on marriage, e.g. Question 109:

Some people say a deaf child needs more smacking than a hearing child, and others say you should try not to smack a deaf child. What do you feel about?

This phrasing allows mothers to reply in either way, knowing that both feelings have been voiced, and that the socially less desirable option is a legitimate one.

In other cases, when asking about the aspects of the child's behaviour that might not be considered so acceptable, the question would imply that this was seen as a real possibility by the interviewer, e.g. Question 66:

Does he make a lot of noise when he eats – this often does seem to be a problem with deaf children?

And Question 92:

I expect he still wets the bed sometimes, doesn't he?

NOTE

1 J. and E. Newson (1963), *Infant Care in an Urban Community* (Allen & Unwin, London).

Appendix III

The Sample

OBTAINING THE SAMPLE

The area chosen for the study was the East Midlands, for our purposes being the counties of Nottinghamshire, Northamptonshire, Leicestershire, Lincolnshire and Derbyshire. This area includes large cities such as Nottingham, Leicester and Derby, large and small towns, villages, and very rural areas in parts of Lincolnshire and Derbyshire.

Local Authorities are required to keep lists of the handicapped children in their area from the age of 2, and this includes children with a hearing loss. It was hoped that the lists maintained by Local Authorities would be relatively complete, as routine screening for deafness in the early months is recognised as a desirable routine policy.

The Medical Officer of Health in each Authority was requested to supply a list of deaf children in his area. Some Authorities felt able to provide a list. Some Authorities had a policy of not supplying lists of children in this way but they were able to co-operate with us by sending out letters from us to the parents with a pre-paid reply to us, allowing those parents who were prepared to be interviewed to contact us.

Our contact rate for the two groups varied as might be expected. Of the eighty-seven names that were provided:

- 62 were interviewed
- 12 had moved from the address given and their new address was not known
- 5 were no longer diagnosed as deaf
- 2 were too old for this study

1 family did not speak English
1 child was in a children's home
1 child diagnosed as aphasic rather than deaf; the mother of
  this child was interviewed but the interview is not included in
  this study
1 mother ill in hospital, suffering from depression
1 mother I was unable to contact despite two letters and two
  visits to the home, when she was out both times
1 outright refusal, on the grounds that the mother had been
  interviewed eight times already.

The non-contact is to all intents and purposes a refusal, and thus
effectively there are two refusals in this group.

From those Authorities who sent out the letters themselves,
seventy-nine letters were sent out. There were forty-nine replies
(61 per cent). Forty-six of the mothers who replied were interviewed,
one mother replied that her child was not now considered to be
deaf, one mother replied and refused, one mother replied saying she
was willing to be interviewed but was found to be out on three pre-
arranged visits to her home. This can also be considered a refusal,
giving two direct refusals in this group.

Of the remaining thirty letters, five were returned as the families
had moved away.

This leaves twenty-five children unaccounted for. Some of the
twenty-five who did not reply can be considered refusals, but going
on the experience of the previous group where names were supplied
and the families who did not reply were visited, this twenty-five
will include:

(i) Some who have moved away, but letters not returned.
(ii) Some children not now diagnosed as deaf
(iii) Some families who do not speak English

Overall one might break the group down into:

108 interviews
4 refusals
25 refusal/non-contact
giving an actual refusal rate of between 3 and 21 per cent.

Further to these 108 interviews in the initial stages of the research,
fourteen interviews were carried out in order to pilot the question-
naire. There were two pilots.

Pilot I in the Nottingham area involved eight mothers of 6-year-old deaf children just outside the range of the main study. After slight modifications, Pilot II was carried out in an area outside the East Midlands of children in the relevant age group. The names of these children were provided by teachers of the deaf and welfare officers in the area. As only slight modifications, mostly in terms of the order of the questions, were made in the interview schedule at the pilot stage, the results of these interviews have been included in the final analysis.

THE INITIAL CONTACT

In those cases where the names and addresses were available, letters were written to the mothers explaining the nature of the research and suggested a time for a visit. Unless arrangements were made to the contrary, the interviewer called at this time to conduct the interview.

In the cases where the letter was sent out by the local Medical Officers of Health, a stamped addressed envelope was enclosed for the parents' reply, together with a form on which they could indicate suitable times for the interviewer to call. The interviewer then replied, making a definite arrangement to call.

THE SAMPLE

The Children
Of the 122 mothers interviewed, seventy two (59 per cent) were mothers of boys and fifty (41 per cent) were mothers of girls.
By age, this was as shown in Table A.1.

Under 2 years	5% (6)
2–3·5 years	25% (31)
3·6–4·11 years	39% (47)
5·0+ years[a]	31% (38)

Table A.1   Age of sample

[a] This includes nine children of 6 and over – eight from the initial pilot and one from the main sample who, though 5 at time of initial contact, was 6 before the actual interview took place.

Social Class
The Registrar General's classification of occupations (1960) was used to classify the families into social class, with two slight modifi-

cations following the Newsons' study of normal children.[1] These were to group Classes I–II into one class, and to divide Class III into two classes (III white collar and III manual), thus distinguishing between the white collar and supervisory manual occupations from the skilled manual. Furthermore, in two cases the family status was upgraded on the strength of the mother's occupational qualifications. This procedure was also followed by Newson and Newson.[2]

Class I–II	32% (39)
Class III WC	11% (14)
Class III M	37% (45)
Class IV	13% (16)
Class V	7% (8)[a]

Table A.2   Class distribution of sample

[a] This distribution remains the same if immigrants and/or the pilot group are excluded.

This in fact shows a much greater number of Class I–II than the normal distribution for the population and differs from the sample studied by the Newsons in this respect.

	I–II	III WC	III M	IV	V
Newsons' sample[a]	14%	13%	50%	15%	8%
This sample	32%	11%	37%	13%	7%

Table A.3   Comparison of class distribution of this sample and a sample of normal 4-year-olds

[a] J. and E. Newson (1968).

There is no immediate and obvious answer as to why there should be such a difference. Deafness does not appear to be any respecter of social class. A major study of children born in the week 3–9 March 1958 found that 'the observed number in each social class did not differ from the expected number'.[3]

There are two factors in the actual sampling that could be operating here. Firstly, the non-replies in the group where the onus was on the parent to make the contact with us could be of a lower class.

A further possibility is that Social Class I–II parents are more likely to suspect deafness in their children and to push to get it diagnosed. In many cases, despite parental concern, early diagnosis was not obtained (see Chapter 7).

The sample includes fourteen immigrant children, 11 per cent of the total sample. They are, in fact, underpresented, for in some cases the house was visited but language difficulties made it impossible to proceed with the interview.

Parents of the children

Most of the children came from normal two-parent families, though two of the children were being brought up by mothers alone. In one of these cases the mother was a widow, in the other she was separated from the child's father. There was also one unmarried mother, but she was living with the child's father, who was acting in all respects as the father of the child.

There were four cases in which children were not being brought up by their natural parents. Two of these children were adopted, one was being fostered on a permanent basis and one was being brought up by the father's sister and her husband because of the break-up of the marriage of the parents.

There were a further four cases in which the acting father was not the natural father of the child. Three of these were mothers divorced from the father of the child who had re-married, and one was a mother, unmarried at the birth of the child, who had later married a man not the child's father.

There was only one case of a child being brought up by the natural father and a stepmother, this again being due to the breakdown of the marriage of the child's natural parents.

Most of the fathers were in occupations that did not take them away from home overnight. One was away two nights a week, one was away three nights a week, ten were away occasionally. Only three were in occupations which meant they normally worked away from home.

A quarter (30) of the fathers were involved in shift work and for twenty-three of these this entailed working some nights.

	Deaf	Normal 4-year-olds
Never	71% (86)	72%
Part-time at home	4% (5)	4%
Full-time at home	2% (3)	1%
Part-time out	16% (20)	19%
Full-time out	7% (8)	4%

Table A.4 Mothers working: a comparison of mothers of deaf and handicapped children

As can be seen from Table A.4, just over a quarter of the mothers were engaged in paid employment, the majority working just part-time. The amount the mothers of deaf children worked was very similar to that of normal 4-year-olds.

In most cases where the mother was working, and in all cases where she was working full-time, the child was at school. In a few cases a relation looked after the child while the mother worked, and in a few others the mother worked a twilight shift, i.e. she worked in the evening, and the child was left with the father, or more occasionally older children.

Age of Parents

Most mothers fell in the 20–27 age group (48 per cent) and most fathers in the 28–35 age group (49 per cent). Only 2 per cent (3) of the mothers were over 44 years at the time of the interview.

Family Size

The majority of children (nearly 60 per cent) came from one- or two-children families, and the vast majority from families of three or less children (80 per cent). Only 6 per cent came from families of five or more children. Thirty children (25 per cent) were eldest children. There were fifty-seven last-born or singletons (47 per cent). It is clearly not possible to make statements on patterns of child-bearing due to having a deaf child based on this data. The data is not comparable with that of the 4-year-old sample, for clearly age makes a difference. This issue is, however, discussed in Chapter 8, where the attitude of parents of a deaf child to having more children is considered.

Twelve of the children had siblings who were also handicapped in some ways. In ten of these (8 per cent of the total sample) the handicap was deafness. Of the other two, one was a child with spina bifida, the other a child who was blind.

Most households comprised only the nuclear family, mother, father and the child or children. In only ten cases were other people living in the house, and in nine of these cases the person was a close relative.

In general, thus, we have 122 ordinary families, some large, some small. On no count would they seem to differ from families in the community at large except for one essential feature, the reason for which we have singled them out – that in all these families there is a deaf child.

NOTES

1 J. and E. Newson (1963, 1968).
2 J. and E. Newson, op. cit.
3 C. S. Peckham, M. Sheridan and N. R. Butler (1972), 'School attainment of seven year old children with hearing difficulties', *Dev. Med. and Child Neurol.*, Vol. 14, No. 5.

Bibliography

Action Research for the Crippled Child (1973), *Does He Take Sugar In His Tea?*

British Deaf and Dumb Association (1970), Report by the Working Party of the BDDA Association formed to study and comment on 'The Lewis Report', published by the BDDA Carlisle

Cook-Gumperz, J. (1973), *Social Control and Socialisations* (Routledge & Kegan Paul, London)

Denmark, J. (1973), 'The education of deaf children', *Hearing*, Vol. 28, No. 9

Ewing, A. W. G. (ed.) (1957), *Educational Guidance and the Deaf Child* (Manchester University Press, Manchester)

Hewett, S. (1970), *The Family and the Handicapped Child* (Allen & Unwin, London)

HMSO (1962), *Handicapped Pupils and Special Schools, Amending Regulations*, Statutory Instrument No. 2073

HMSO (1968), *The Education of Deaf Children* (Department of Education and Science, London)

HMSO (1969), *Peripatetic Teachers of the Deaf, Education Survey 6* (Department of Education and Science, London)

John, J. E. J. (1964), 'Hearing aids', in A. and E. C. Ewing, *Teaching Deaf Children to Talk* (Manchester University Press, Manchester)

John Tracy Clinic, *Correspondence Course for Parents of Pre-school Deaf Children* (1968), available from John Tracy Clinic, 806 West Adams Boulevard, Los Angeles, California 90007

Keller, H. (1902), *The Story of My Life* (Doubleday, New York)

Kendall, D. C. (1953), 'The mental development of young deaf children', unpublished PhD thesis (University of Manchester, Manchester)

Lewis, M. M. (1963), *Language, Thought and Personality in Infancy and Childhood* (Harrap, London)

Ling, A. H. (1968) 'Advice for parents of young deaf children: how to begin', *Review*, Vol. 12, No. 70

Meadow, K. P. (1966), 'Early manual communication in relation to the child's intellectual, social and communicative functioning', *American Annals of the Deaf*, No. 113

Meadow, K. P. (1967), 'The effect of early manual communication and family climate on the deaf child's development', unpublished PhD dissertation (University of California, Berkeley)

Newson, J. and E. (1963), *Infant Care in an Urban Community* (Allen & Unwin, London)

Newson, J. and E. (1968), *Four Years Old in an Urban Community* (Allen & Unwin, London)

Newson, J. and E. (undated), *What Is an Autistic Child?* (prepared for the Nottingham and District Society for Autistic Children)

Peckham, C. S., Sheridan, M. and Butler, N. R. (1972), 'School attainment of seven year old children with hearing difficulties', *Dev. Med. and Child Neurol.*, Vol. 14, No. 5

Quigley, S. P. (1969), *The Influence of Finger Spelling on the Development of Language Communication, and Educational Achievements of Deaf Children* (Institute for Research into Exceptional Children, University of Illinois)

Royal National Institute for the Deaf (1968), *Conversation with the Deaf*, 8th edn.

Schlesinger, H. S. and Meadow, K. P. (1972), *Sound and Sign: Childhood Deafness and Mental Health* (University of California Press, Berkeley)

Smith, Gordon (1970), *Points for Speakers about Deaf Children* (National Deaf Children's Society publication)

Spock, B. (1966), *Baby and Child Care* (English edition) (The New English Library, London)

Stuckless, E. R. and Birch, J. W. (1966), 'The influence of early manual communication on the linguistic development of deaf children', *American Annals of the Deaf*, No. III

Svendsen, M. (1934), 'Children's imaginary companions', *Archives of Neurology and Psychiatry*, No. 32

Thames Television production (1973), 'Sunday and Monday in Silence'

Williams, K. M. (1972), *You Can Help Your Deaf Child* (National College for Teachers of the Deaf)

Wood, H. C. (1970), 'Problems in the development and home care of pre-school blind children', unpublished PhD thesis (University of Nottingham)

Wright, E. (1972), *The New Childhood* (Tandem Books, London)

Index